Health Information Science

Series Editor

Yanchun Zhang

More information about this series at http://www.springer.com/series/11944

Kerstin Denecke

Health Web Science

Social Media Data for Healthcare

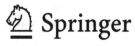 Springer

Kerstin Denecke
Innovation Center for Computer Assisted Surgery
Universität Leipzig
Leipzig, Sachsen, Germany

Health Information Science
ISBN 978-3-319-35223-7   ISBN 978-3-319-20582-3   (eBook)
DOI 10.1007/978-3-319-20582-3

Springer Cham Heidelberg New York Dordrecht London

Printed on acid-free paper

Springer International Publishing AG Switzerland is part of Springer Science+Business Media (www.
springer.com)

"In the past, we went to the medical doctor (Dr. med.) when we became sick. Today, we are asking Dr. Google."

Preface

The web became a rich source of personal information during the last years. People are twittering, blogging and chatting online. Feelings, experiences or latest news are posted everywhere in the web. Face-to-face communication seems to be replaced or at least extended by the new communication tools. Since this new communication style provides insights into thoughts of individuals and their behaviour, reflects trends and situations in the real world, it became focus of research, politics and economics. For instance, first hints to disease outbreaks or political changes can be identified from this data. Beyond, companies discover the benefits of analysing social web communication for developing and adapting marketing strategies.

The developments of the web and mobile communications led to the rise of a new research field summarized under the term *Web Science*. What is Web Science and more specifically, what characterizes Health Web Science—the topic of this book?

The American computer scientist Ben Shneiderman claims that "Web Science" is a "new way of thinking about computer science" [1]. Tim Berners-Lee becomes more specific: "Web Science must be inherently interdisciplinary; its goal is both, to understand the growth of the web and to create approaches that allow new powerful and more beneficial patterns to occur" [2]. For short, not only processing the information available on the web is part of the Web Science research agenda, but also social issues such as trust, reputation and privacy play an important role. Starting from this understanding, we define *Health Web Science* as follows:

Health Web Science is the medico-socio-technical science that investigates how the web evolves with respect to health issues, how health related data provided through the web can be processed and how tools that make use of web technology can be used in healthcare.

In other words, Health Web Science is about patients, doctors and health carers, the information they are providing in the web, the tools they can use to communicate on health issues and about methods to support in analysing the provided health information. Health Web Science targets at understanding how the web shapes and is shaped by medicine, healthcare and people, and how the web interacts and impacts on health [3].

With an increased interest in e-Health, Health 2.0, Medicine 2.0 and the recent birth of the discipline of Web Science, this book targets at introducing the field of Health Web Science with its facets in use cases and at presenting methods for gathering information from written medical social media data. How these methods can be exploited for social media analysis will be shown through example applications. The influence factors discussed at the end of the book serve as entry point for future developments in research and discussion.

This book is the result of my research activities at the L3S Research Center in Hannover and at the Innovation Center for Computer Assisted Surgery in Leipzig. Collaborations with colleagues in the EU-funded research projects LivingKnowledge and M-Eco motivated to dig into depth of this extremely interesting field of Health Web Science. Thanks to Yihan Deng who provided code to analyse linguistic characteristics in Chap. 6. The work presented in Chap. 11 is a result of the work of the M-Eco consortium whom I would like to thank for the interesting collaboration. Beyond, I would like to thank the members of the IMIA Social Media Working group who provide a very productive platform for discussion and joint research. Last but not least, I would like to thank my friends and family for support on multiple levels as well as for many valuable suggestions for improving the presentation in this book.

Braunschweig, Germany   Kerstin Denecke
April 2015

Contents

Part V   Influence Factors

Part I
Introduction

During the last years, social media started to become prevalent in the context of medicine and health. Medicine 2.0, e-Medicine and Dr. Google are changing dramatically the healthcare system. Each patient can become his personal doctor: The web provides tools for self-diagnosis, for self-monitoring, information on treatment options. It is representing a platform for self-help where people suffering from diseases receive information and support from others. Clearly, medical social media content exchanged and communicated through the web differs from the information in the "normal" web: Persons report about the most precious and private issue they possess which is their life and their health. They describe their personal destiny, diseases and symptoms they are experiencing. Success or failures of the medical treatments and drugs are discussed; experiences in living with medical conditions are reflected. This makes the medical web content a source of very personal information (Fig. 1).

A big question is: How can healthcare benefit from the millions of web pages and the broad range of social media tools and data? How to analyse the available data? As a motivation, this part of the book provides insights into the possibilities, social media can provide to healthcare. Starting with a brief overview on the authors of medical social media, their information needs and the content they are providing in the web, we will closer look at concrete application areas. Various web technologies that are already supporting or could support in near future in healthcare processes will be introduced.

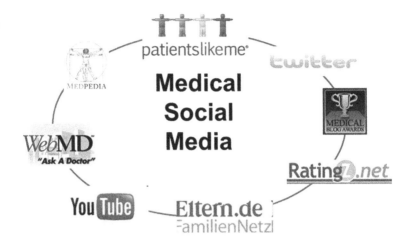

Fig. 1 Facets of the medical web: social networks, microblogging sites, blog pages, forums, wikis, rating portals and others form the medical web

Chapter 1
The Medical Web and Its Authors

1.1 What is Medical Social Media?

The advances in Internet and mobile technologies changed the way how people access, use and share information. Social media tools arose and now provide manifold opportunities to share information or encourage social networking and communication [4]. **Social media** are digital media and technologies that enable users to exchange information and to create media content on their own or in community with others. Data and experiences are distributed via social media tools such as instant messaging, blogs, social networking (e.g. Facebook) or video sharing (e.g. YouTube). They opened new ways of communicating and enabled for timeless and location-independent information exchange.

Individuals are engaged by social media in one-to-many conversations using electronic communication tools. The term "social media" is used to refer to both, the underlying technologies such as forums or blogs and to the data, the text, images or whatever content that is provided through such tools in the web and shared with others.

Social media data includes various kinds of publicly available content that is produced by end-users, rather than by the operator of a web site. Often, content has been uploaded without a commercial, marketing or promotional purpose in mind. However, also companies or organisations are increasingly using social media for promoting products and services.

Medical social media data is a subset of the social media data space, in which the interests of the participants are specifically devoted to medicine and health issues. More specifically, with **medical social media data** we refer to web-based narrative text that contains some medical content which was written by individuals (potential patients), physicians or other healthcare professionals. In general, the content in medical social media is characterized by a mixture of expert knowledge, layman knowledge or experiences and empirical findings [5]. Blogs with primary topics related to medicine or health care are considered medical blogs. Medical blogs

© Springer International Publishing Switzerland 2015
K. Denecke, *Health Web Science*, Health Information Science,
DOI 10.1007/978-3-319-20582-3_1

constitute an important part of the public medium of medicine because they offer novel channels that reach a wider range of medical audiences and provide new avenues for medical bloggers to disseminate health-related information [6].

Which information and tools are available and how can patients and health carers benefit? What characterises the medical web? In general, the **medical web** consists of social media tools and data provided through these tools (see Chap. 4). This book focuses on the automatic processing of the content or data provided though social media tools. This content comprises data and information on diseases, treatments, drugs, experiences and best practices provided by different authors having various intentions in mind. Thus, the authors of medical web contributions can be individuals or organizations. Individuals are single patients, physicians or health carers. Organizations comprise hospitals, companies from the healthcare industry, health organizations, health insurances.

1.2   Personas

Eysenbach [7] identified three main personas (user groups and content provider) of Web 2.0 applications in health care: patients, health professionals, and biomedical researchers. These persona provide evidence-based or experiential information on diseases, treatments, and medications from their perspectives.

Health professionals treat patients either as physician, as nurse, as physiotherapist, etc. They are using the medical web (1) to share their practical knowledge and skills. Examples of such blogs include CasesBlog [8] or KevinMD [9]. (2) Health professionals in turn search for information in the medical web. They can learn from the experiences of their colleagues provided through social media platforms such as blogs or fora or can access latest results from clinical research. (3) Health professionals provide information through the web. For example, medical centres inform in their YouTube channels on latest research achievements in clinical therapy (e.g. the YouTube channel of the Mayo clinic [10]). The Mayo Clinic Center for Social Media compiled a list of health-related organisations that are actively using social networking sites [11]. It shows that healthcare providers become increasingly aware of the new possibilities of the web to provide health information and share them with patients. Additionally, health professionals (4) interact with patients through social media. Information can be exchanged; the patient's health can be monitored etc. Thus, health professionals interact with other individuals or groups of this persona type or with patients. As artefacts, they are providing texts in blogs, forums, wikis or even multimedia content in form of podcasts or videos. They need information on diseases, clinical evidences, experiences of their colleagues and patient health data in order to comply their professional tasks.

The persona **patient** is a person who is suffering from symptoms or a disease, but can also be a relative or friend of a sick person. Fox et al. [12] identified three patient user groups: the well, the acute and the chronic. While the "well" are searching seldom for health information and focus on information on prevention mainly, the "acute" are the most active searchers in the medical web. The "chronic" use social media for managing their disease. The patients use blogs to share their own health and disease experiences [13, 14]. Beyond, patients increasingly rely on the web when looking for medical information and advice. A survey performed by the Pew Research Center and California Healthcare foundation found out that 66 % of Internet users look online for information about a specific disease or medical problem and 56 % search for information on a particular treatment [12]. Even the elderly use the Internet to search for health information [15]. Further, patients communicate and interact with their health professionals, asking questions, or send measured values for monitoring purposes. As artefacts, they are providing texts in blogs, forums, wikis or even multimedia content in form of podcasts or videos. They search for information on diseases, treatments and drugs including ratings and experiences from other patients. Additionally, they are providing health data to health professionals.

The persona **biomedical researcher** exploit medical social media on the one hand to provide research results. Even more interestingly is the use of medical social media for analysis purposes such as predicting disease outbreaks [16], patient recruitment or analysing treatment outcomes. This persona needs aggregated information on disease or symptom mentions, on efficacy of drugs and treatments. Beyond, they require facilities to search for groups of patients with specific characteristics (for patient recruitment). As artefacts, they are reporting about clinical studies or research results in blogs, forums, or wikis.

Table 1.1 summarises personas of the medical web in terms of their information needs and their information provided in the web. In Sect. 6.1, example blogs from physicians and patients are compared with respect to their content, giving more detailed insights into data provided through social media tools.

Table 1.1 Personas of the medical web, examples of their information needs and content provided

Persona	Information and content need	Information provided	Interacts with
Patient	Information on diseases, treatment, prevention, management tools for diseases	Personal health information, experiences with treatments and diseases	Health professional, other patients
Healthcare professional	Best practices, latest research results	Evidence-based or experiential knowledge about diseases, treatment, medications	Other health professionals, patients
Researcher	Treatment outcomes, information on disease development and progression	Research results	Other researchers

Chapter 2
Applications of Social Media in Healthcare

Web technologies and social media exist already for several years and are increasingly exploited to support in healthcare processes. One cannot ignore the fact that social media has already dramatically changed the structure of healthcare delivery in the modern world. Mayo Clinic researchers have opined that social media has begun a process of "revolutionizing healthcare" by improving healthcare and quality of life [17]. User-generated content on the web has become a new source of useful information to be added to the conventional methods of collecting clinical data. Beyond, web technologies allow for new possibilities in collaboration and information exchange in healthcare.

Mainly two groups of social media applications in healthcare can be distinguished: One group of applications is centred around social media tools and web technologies, that are exploited for healthcare purposes. A second group of applications is centred around the analysis of (medical) social media data. More specifically, medical social media tools and web technologies can be exploited in healthcare for:

1. Supporting the treatment process (Sect. 2.1),
2. Preventing diseases, promoting health activity, supporting in disease self assessment (Sect. 2.2),
3. Networking, gathering and exchanging of health information (Sect. 2.3), or for
4. Managing medical knowledge (Sect. 2.4).

The data available in the web provided through social media tools can additionally be used to support in healthcare processes among others by extending clinical data or making the data available for (clinical) research and health monitoring purposes (Sect. 2.5).

In the following, application areas and corresponding use cases of the above mentioned categories are described with the purpose of highlighting the technical challenges and requirements for their realisation. The described applications are either already in practical use or demonstrate future scenarios. Each section

© Springer International Publishing Switzerland 2015
K. Denecke, *Health Web Science*, Health Information Science,
DOI 10.1007/978-3-319-20582-3_2

ends with a description of the—mainly technical—requirements for realising the applications. Table 2.2 at the end of the chapter summarizes the application areas and requirements.

2.1 Social Media Support for Patient Treatment

During a treatment process many interactions between a patient, a physician or other healthcare provider take place, starting with an initial meeting and examination, followed by diagnosis and interactions after the physician decided for a diagnosis. In a simple case, a patient gets prescribed a medication and he is cured after some days without any additional patient-physician interactions; the patient can even recover at home. For complex or chronic diseases, the treatment process can take several weeks, months or even years during which monitoring of symptoms, treatment successes or of the health status in general is necessary. Several healthcare providers including specialized physicians and therapists are involved in the whole treatment process. Continuous monitoring and patient treatment requires extensive information exchange and communication among involved persons (which so far often does not take place) and a patient needs to see the doctor regularly. Such face-to-face visits are time-consuming for all involved parties, the healthcare team and the patient. Beyond, the communication barriers are high.

Social media and web technologies can be exploited to support in long-term treatment processes. In particular, they can enable a continuous monitoring and self-management of diseases from a patient's perspective. Observations on the health status can be entered by the patient himself, for example through diabetes self-management tools, pain management apps [18], symptom diaries, or apps for glucose level reporting [19]. Consider the following fictitious example, where social media tools support a patient in self-managing his disease.

> George, suffering from chronic pain, keeps regularly an online diary where he records the strength of his pain, its location and other relevant information related to his disease. The diary has some options for free-textual entries, provides pain scales, where George simply has to select a value as well as checkboxes to answer questions. George's physician and healthcare team can access his diary via a secure login. This allows them to monitor the symptoms and health status of George. The questions in the diary are put together by George's physician and his carers. To facilitate the analysis and continuous screening of the diary content, automatic tools pre-filter the content or even analyse it and provide notifications to the physician or other carers automatically when the health status changes according to the diary entries of George.

The example shows: Exploiting social media tools during the treatment process can allow for a continuous, close health monitoring by reducing time-consuming face-to-face visits. Further, social media based collaboration platforms enable patients and health carers to communicate with each other, to regularly report and to exchange information during the treatment process [20]. Online psychological support during treatment or internet-based nurse support can be provided through such platforms. In addition, social media tools can support in realising integrated healthcare processes. The latter often lack of sufficient communication and information exchange among health carers. If at all, the patient is the medium of communication, transporting information, reports and images from one carer to another. A social network-like platform among carers could overcome this lack. All involved carers could stay informed and communicate easily, not only via a patient, but through the platform (which should be of course restricted in access). Even an information exchange with additional actors (e.g. nursing services, therapists) may be enabled through social media technology. This may support in optimizing healthcare processes. Corresponding approaches are already available: AmbulanzPartner (http://www.ambulanzpartner.de) is a social network-like platform that coordinates the healthcare process and all involved persons (patients, physicians, therapists, healthcare provider etc.).

Requirements: Social media based applications supporting patient treatment should provide facilities for entering health data. This data needs only to be accessible to relevant healthcare provider or other persons involved in the treatment process. Clearly, appropriate data privacy and security issues as well as access restrictions need to be implemented. Since the amount of data can become huge, physicians or healthcare provider need support in analysing the data. They should be pointed directly to problems and changes in the health status (e.g. by getting an alert). Data visualisation is crucial in such applications for both, patient and physician, to quickly get an overview on changes in the health status. For the healthcare provider, data access to relevant clinical data or the electronic health record is important to document or adequately judge decisions made. Further, corresponding communication facilities, e.g. message boards or chat rooms need to be integrated for enabling an informal information exchange among carers and with patients.

2.2   Social Media for Preventing Diseases and Promoting Health Activity

Applications are arising where social media is used for disease prevention, i.e. social media supports in guiding and supporting health behaviour. For example, social networking sites are exploited for smoking prevention activities directed specifically towards young women [21]. Physical activity may be triggered and increased through internet-based interventions. The following scenario demonstrates this use case:

Fred, a 49 year-old man suffering from Parkinson's disease accesses through a web portal videos and descriptions of physical activity exercises his therapists prepared and selected particularly for him considering his current health status. The exercises are provided through an individualized online portal to Fred and he performs the activities on an individual basis, but with support of online tutorials or videos provided by the therapists. Fred records once a week the exercises and stores them back to the portal where his carer can access them, can provide feedback, monitor the progress and, in case the health status worsens, ask Fred to come to an appointment via a messaging function built into the portal. Fred can also leave questions or comments for his therapists in the portal reflecting his experiences or difficulties that help the therapists and physician to monitor the health status and to adjust the exercises.

The benefit of online-based health activity programs is that the patient can decide when to exercise. The barriers of making the exercises are reduced since no direct observation by a physician or therapist takes place. At the same time, monitoring and feedback by a health carer is possible after watching videos recorded and provided by the patient while doing an exercise.

Requirements: With respect to health activity promotion using web technologies, facilities for video recording, and indirect communication are necessary. Realising health activity programs as group games requires social gaming technology. Gamification methods, i.e. game thinking and game design elements, can be exploited for increasing the compliance of patients [22]. Facilities for providing feedback and exchanging messages between patients and health carers need to be established. Physicians and therapists need to be enabled to generate and manage therapeutic exercises.

2.3 Social Media Tools for Networking, Information Gathering and Exchange

Hospitals, physicians or other healthcare provider start presenting their health services as well as treatment programs or information on disease prevention on their websites (with varying quality and readability [23]). For example, healthcare providers offer YouTube videos for patient education, (e.g. the Mayo clinic offers educational videos for patients at YouTube [10] on the heart and circulatory system). Physicians keep blogs where they inform patients about vaccination campaigns or new treatment options. Gathering and providing information on diseases, symptoms and treatments is becoming another application of social media, used already frequently by patients [12]. Studies of the Pew Internet Project's research showed a substantial raise of U.S. users who searched in the web for information on medical conditions and treatments: The number of adults who use the internet for health information retrieval increased from 72 % in 2012 to 87 % in 2014 [24].

Information search and access through the internet supports patient empowerment, resulting increasingly in "expert patients" [25]. One of the most active groups of online health-information seekers are those who suffer from chronic conditions or from rare diseases [26]. By surfing in cyberspace, patients can learn what others have to say about quality of care, or about important issues regarding treatment and diagnosis. In addition to gaining knowledge, online medical-information seekers are able to communicate with other persons who are suffering from the same disease which helps in reducing feelings of isolation and loneliness. The following scenario describes information exchange through social media tools:

Fred, who is using the online activity program (see scenario in the previous section), connects to other patients with Parkinson's disease via a platform and online message board. He receives through this platform information on scheduled meetings of the self-help group and interesting information posted by others. From time to time, he posts his experiences with the activity games or asks other patients for their experiences with the disease. Once a week, an online chat is organised where sometimes healthcare providers are invited to join the chat and answer the questions of the group on specific topics. In this way, Fred learns more about his disease and gets in contact with other persons suffering from the same medical condition. In particular, when his health status worsens, he gets support by other network participants. He benefits from their experiences in dealing with his disease.

One distinct advantage offered by medical social media communication is that the communication barriers are considerably lower than for face-to-face communication [27]. This may allow patients to write on social media platforms more freely about their illnesses and their experiences with drugs and medical treatments than they would normally do in other settings. Personal experiences and opinions on health issues are shared with others who have the same health concerns already comprehensively through platforms like E-Patient-Dave or PatientsLikeMe. With social media, self-help received a new dimension: Patients can interact and communicate with each other over long distances, even if they cannot move from home. There are online patient communities that organise themselves, i.e. content is exchanged without any support or interaction of healthcare providers. Other patient networks are upcoming that are explicitly designed for patient education or allow for interactions with physicians (e.g. an online support group for depression [28]). Social networks enable patients to actively take care of their health. They can exchange information on symptoms, therapies, medications, treatment alternatives or can get in contact with experts or self-help groups. Some additional usage scenarios are listed below (Table 2.1).

Table 2.1 Usage scenarios for social networks

Scenario	Example network platforms
Single users provide healthcare information, e.g. in their blogs	http://www.epatients.net, www.thehealthcareblog.com
Patients connect to each other and communicate in patient communities	http://www.patientslikeme. com, http://www. iwantgreatcare.org
Patients exchange their health care data anonymously and generate in this way disease-related knowledge databases	http://www.curetogether.com
Patients communicate with doctors	http://www.paginemediche.it
Doctors communicate with each other in unspecific or interdisciplinary platforms	http://www.doctors.net.uk, http://www.sermo.com, www.medting.com
Doctors communicate in subfield-specific fora	http://www.neurosurgic.com
Doctors communicate in general health portals	http://www.imedo.de
Doctors communicate in topic-specific communities	http://www.acor.org

Additionally, healthcare provider may exploit networking platforms for exchanging their experiences on the treatment and healthcare process (e.g. DocsBoard [29]) or get latest research results by going through the information provided by their colleagues. Beyond, they can use social networking to crowdsource answers to clinical questions.

Requirements: For information gathering applications, corresponding search facilities are required—the available amount of information is huge and in particular for patients, it is difficult to formulate adequate queries and to select high-quality result pages. Therefore, search facilities need to support different user groups in query formulation. Given the large variety of available health information in the web, it is also important to provide users means for judging the quality of web content. Extremely important in this context are quality measures (e.g. HONcode [30]) that allow users to judge the reliability of some information. To realise applications for networking and information exchange, no particular requirements are to be fulfilled from a technical perspective. Corresponding facilities for social networks or forums are sufficient and simply need to be implemented with adequate access rights. When social network technology is used for connecting healthcare provider and patient data is exchanged through this channel, ethical issues, data privacy and security issues need to be considered (see Chap. 14).

2.4 Social Media Tools for Managing Knowledge

Another field of application of social media is knowledge management within medical or clinical research and science. Departments, research consortia etc. are using collaborative writing tools such as wikis or Google documents for making knowledge available or for managing knowledge [31]. Social media can further provide a tool for collecting experiences on treatments made by physicians. Detailed knowledge can be made available in wikis or other social media platforms among others for educational purposes or for exchanging experiences. For example surgical transcripts were collaboratively collected at Wikisurgery (the website was taken offline in 2012) as an information repository on best surgical practice. Consider the following scenario:

> Dr. Harris is neurologist and specialised on treatment of patients with multiple sclerosis. There is a lot of research on this disease ongoing. He regularly posts his experiences with treatment options and on latest research results he became aware of, on a wiki dealing specifically with treatment of multiple sclerosis. Only physicians are allowed to contribute to this wiki. Dr. Harris also checks the entries from others and learns more about their experiences and new treatment options. In this way, he and his colleagues exchange experiences and knowledge and stay up to date.

The scenario shows: Social media technology has the potential of supporting physicians in retrieving best practices and accordingly, in making treatment decision following the latest clinical evidences. A clinical trial[1] was run at the University of Texas Health Science Center at Houston targeting at improving surgical residents' skills in critically appraising the literature and to promote the dissemination and application of the best available evidence to surgical practice. The study confirmed the hypothesis that mandatory participation with faculty oversight, in a journal club wiki improves the dissemination, evaluation, and application of evidence-based medicine.

Collaborative writing is also possible for patient communities (e.g. a wiki with patient experiences on drugs or treatments), but such applications are still rare. An example is the service *Patient Opinion* [32], a platform that collects experiences from patients to improve healthcare.

Requirements: Knowledge management applications require corresponding technologies, i.e. wikis, or document sharing facilities for managing knowledge by means of web technologies. A very important, but non-technical issue is that people are actively contributing content to those applications. In particular wikis require continuous updates and extensions to be useful sources of information.

2.5   Research and Health Monitoring Using Social Media Data

Beyond, social media content becomes also more and more subject of research and monitoring in healthcare and medicine. Instead of using the social media tools for healthcare purposes as described in the applications and scenarios presented before, medical social media data, i.e. textual data provided through web technologies, is analysed and interpreted for monitoring and research purposes even more intensively.

The motivation behind grounds among others upon the fact that social media data provides a new information source for researchers to learn about experiences of patients (and of physicians). Feelings, perceptions, experiences are often unconsidered in the treatment process given the short amount of contact time between a physician and a patient. Experiences of patients with respect to treatments and drugs reported in social media can be analysed for studying efficiency of treatments or treatment preferences; risks provoked by drugs can be identified from patient case data provided online for the purpose of pharmaceutical research. There is for example Treato.com, a social health site that analyses online patient discussions to provide insights from patients' opinions and attitudes, helping to answer questions about a medication. Through the study of social media data, for example of illness

---

[1]Clinical study: Use of Wikis and Evidence-Based Medicine in Surgical Practice, ClinicalTrials.gov Identifier: NCT01051050, completed in 2011, http://clinicaltrials.gov/\discretionary-show/\discretionary-NCT01051050.

narratives, healthcare providers and the research community can learn how and what patients wish to share with their online health community, how patients view their illness and treatment, and which gaps or successes in treatment patients recognise [33].

Further, medical social media data provides new research possibilities and insights for example into the course of therapy from a patient's and physician's perspective. A large amount of information on patient behaviour, i.e. patient experiences on treatments and drugs is available in the web, ready to be used for research and studies. For example the web portal "Ask a Patient" [34] provides drug reviews describing side effects that occurred while taking a specific medication. There are many research questions that can be addressed when analysing medical social media data. The information provided through this channel is unique in a sense that there is no other written source of experiences from patients and health carers.

Another application area in this context is the recruitment of patients for clinical trials based on their social media profiles or exploitation of social media data for epidemiological studies [35]. Further, potential health risks can be identified based on social media data and a population's health status can be monitored [36] (see Sect. 11).

Requirements: Technically, a broad range of methods is necessary to realise monitoring and analysis of medical social media data. Web content needs to be collected and filtered according to its relevance to a research question. For analysing the social media data, methods are required for:

- Crawling web data,
- Filtering or classifying,
- Textmining, extracting information, mapping to ontologies,
- Statistical analysis,
- Search and retrieval,
- Integrating with clinical data and
- Visualization.

Table 2.2 Categories of social media applications in healthcare, their characterization and technical requirements

Application purpose	Description	Technical requirements
Support of treatment process	**What?** Support of information exchange and communication	Text mining, integration with clinical data, methods for data visualisation, data entry, communication, consideration of privacy and security
	Who? Healthcare provider, patient	
	Why? Closer monitoring, reduce face-to-face consultations (increase independence of patient), ensure continuous care	
	How? Keeping online diaries, exploiting self-management tools, using exchange and collaboration platforms	
Disease prevention, health activity promotion	**What?** Health activity programs	Video recording and management tools, support in communication, and information exchange, social gaming technology
	Who? Healthcare provider, patient	
	Why? Exercising time and location independent, self-motivation, patient empowerment, making exercises in private environment helps acting more freely	
	How? Providing exercises by therapists, recording of exercising activity of patients	
Networking, information exchange and gathering	**What?** Exchanging experiences and knowledge with other patients or carers, information provision and search	Networking platforms, retrieval methods, visualization, quality measures
	Who? Healthcare provider, patient	
	Why? Psychological support, receiving expertise from others	
	How? Using social networking sites, discussion boards, chat rooms	

(continued)

Table 2.2 (continued)

Application purpose	Description	Technical requirements
Knowledge management	**What?** Sharing information	Document sharing technology, methods for formalising knowledge
	Who? Researchers	
	Why? Easy access, generate content collaboratively	
	How? Providing content in wikis, blogs	
Research and monitoring	**What?** Monitoring health behaviour or population health, experiences, opinions, learn about experienced outcomes of treatments and medications	Web crawling, methods for text mining, natural language processing, filtering, statistical analysis, data mining, visualisation, search and retrieval, integration with clinical data
	Who? Researcher, health organisations	
	Why? Rich source of subjective information, timeliness	
	How? Mining data provided via social media tools	

Chapter 3
Objectives and Structure of the Book

In the previous sections, we described applications of social media tools and web technologies as well as usage scenarios for social media data in healthcare. It became clear that the main potentials in this area are

1. Provision of time- and location-independent support,
2. Simplification and support of communication and information exchange,
3. Participation of patients in decision making processes,
4. Patient empowerment through information gathering facilities,
5. Integrated healthcare processes,
6. New research and health monitoring possibilities.

Social media allows to shift information gathering, communication and health monitoring from the social and healthcare sector into the private environment. It thus allows for a location-independent support, can increase the personal convenience and helps in preserving personal independence by simultaneously enabling continuous monitoring. A better risk awareness can be achieved [16]. Social media provides also new possibilities for healthcare prevention, for example through enabling continuous health status monitoring for patients and health carers, or through motivation to do health activities using social games.

3.1 Objectives

From the use cases and applications described before, we derived requirements and technical components necessary for the realisation of the scenarios (see also Table 2.2). In this book, we focus on applications that are exploiting the health-related web data and resist on going into more detail with applications that use social media technology to support healthcare. The main objective is to introduce methods necessary to realise scenarios that are related to information retrieval,

K. Denecke, *Health Web Science*, Health Information Science,
DOI 10.1007/978-3-319-20582-3_3

health data analysis and health care monitoring (i.e. scenarios as described in Sects. 2.3 and 2.5). Since the realisation of such scenarios often requires similar groups of methods, an architecture will be presented for building applications that exploit medical social media data. Despite these constraints in the focus of the book, the methods introduced herein are necessary also for supporting in the other scenarios described.

Our main objective is achieved through focusing on two sub-goals:

1. Introducing methods for processing and analysing medical social media data, and
2. Collecting technical, legal and ethical aspects to be considered when social media data is exploited in healthcare.

To achieve objective 1, we will introduce methods for concept mapping, relation extraction, sentiment analysis and information retrieval. The methods base upon algorithms from machine learning and computer linguistics and have been specifically developed to deal with the characteristics of medical social media data. Content and language of medical social media data will be studied by means of an empirical analysis to collect these characteristics. To achieve objective 2, we will collect legal and ethical aspects that need to be considered when implementing social media into healthcare processes. These aspects have been collected through discussions with experts and a literature review.

3.2   Research Questions and Structure of the Book

This book considers multiple research questions (see Fig. 3.1).

- Theoretical questions about the nature of medical social media data, i.e.

    - What characterises medical social media in terms of content, types, language and structure?

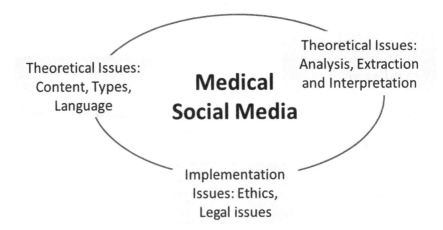

Fig. 3.1 Medical social media: objectives and research questions addressed in this book

– What differences in content and language exist compared to clinical documents?

• Theoretical questions about analysing social media data

– To what extent are (clinical) information extraction tools suited for analysing medical social media texts?
– Which methods can help to extract relations among medical concepts?
– How to assess and provide information on content diversity to a user?

• Practical questions of implementing social media in healthcare, i.e.

– Which ethical and legal question are relevant in this context?

Answering these questions is crucial to understand medical social media, the benefits and limitations of its usage and exploitation in healthcare and to develop methods to realise corresponding applications.

Providing information using web technologies or social media tools is one side of the medal. Gathering and analysing the data that is provided and making use of it for healthcare purposes is the other side. We concentrate in this book on the second side. Thus, the focus is on automatic processing of the content of the medical web, since we believe that medical social media data can provide a complement to clinical data in healthcare applications. We started in this part with describing application categories for medical social media and web technologies. Part II sketches the medical web with types of medical social media and describes the language and structure compared to those of clinical documents. At the end, the challenges or requirements for automatic processing are collected. In Part III we are introducing methods for analysing medical social media data, including methods for concept mapping, relation extraction and sentiment analysis. Examples for applications and their realisation will be highlighted in Part IV. Finally, there are several factors that influence the application and use of web technologies to support healthcare processes. They will be sketched in Part V of the book.

3.3 Material and Methods

To achieve the objectives of the book, a set of methods is developed or applied to medical social media. Since no medical social media data set is available for research purposes, we established a data set collected from blogs in the web. All datasets used for development and analysis in this book are summarized in Table 3.2 and are described in more detail in the following. Table 3.1 gives an overview on the different chapters and the methods and data sets exploited.

The data set underlying most of the studies comprises a random sample of around 12,800 texts in English collected from 65 blogs over a period of four years starting in 2009 from RSS feeds provided through the blogs. We refer to this data set as "MSM data set". The data set consists of patient- and physician-written blog postings.

Table 3.1 Material and methods used in the different parts of the book for analysis and method development

Task/Topic	Material	Methods	Chapter
Sublanguage analysis	Clinical documents, MSM dataset, drug reviews, Slashdot	POS Tagging, pattern analysis, relation extraction, quantitative analysis of word statistics, POS tagging, lexicon lookup with SentiWordNet, subjectivity lexicon	Chapter 6
Architecture development	–	Requirement analysis, service-oriented architecture design principle	Section 7
Concept mapping	MSM data set	cTakes, MetaMap	Chapter 8
Relation extraction	Surgical reports	OpenIE, rules	Chapter 9
Sentiment analysis	Clinical documents, MSM dataset, drug reviews, Slashdot	Quantitative analysis of word statistics, POS tagging, lexicon lookup with SentiWordNet, subjectivity lexicon	Chapter 10
Diversity-aware search	MSM dataset	Machine learning, MetaMap	Chapter 12
Ethical/Legal questions	–	Questionnaire, literature review	Chapter 14

Two thirds of the collected blogs are provided by health professionals. Only for the content analysis, we also considered patient-written postings. They originated from Stellarlife [37], a blog written by a woman suffering from multiple sclerosis, from the blog of Randy Pausch [38] who was suffering from cancer and from Diabetesmine [39], a blog kept by a journalist suffering from diabetes. It provides a mix of news, views, reviews, guest posts, interviews, videos, cartoons, questions and answers and any other type of content useful for people touched by diabetes.

Physician-written postings originate from the blogs of WebMD [40] and EverydayHealth [41], from the Medicinenet website [42], as well as from other blog sources. WebMD provides health information provided in a blog style by physicians. EverydayHealth.com is a provider of online health information designed for non-health professionals. MedicineNet.com provides authoritative medical information for consumers. The RSS feeds were collected, the URL to the complete text identified and the text extracted from the HTML page.

Additionally, we collected drug reviews from DrugRatingz.com [43]. In drug reviews, users can anonymously rate drugs in several categories including effectiveness, side effects, convenience and value. They can post and read comments. These comments, dealing with symptoms and side effects, provide the data set for our analysis while the ratings remain unconsidered. Drugratingz.com is part of a family of websites dedicated to help consumers in finding the best businesses, places, and services by sharing ratings and reviews. Thousand entries have been gathered from that source.

For comparison reasons, we further considered technical interviews downloaded from the website Slashdot [44]. Slashdot is a technology-related weblog, where users express their opinions on technical topics. We chose the technical interviews as benchmark instead of movie or product review, since technical interviews also contain a relatively large amount of domain-specific terminology. We have chosen this particular dataset from the technical domain since it belongs to the category of user-generated, subjective content. Thousand entries have been gathered from that data source.

Additionally, we created a domain-specific corpus comprising clinical documents (nurse letters, radiology reports and discharge summaries). These documents were collected from the "MIMIC II Database".[1] A nurse letter is part of a patient record, which is written by nurses on duty. Its content comprises observations of the nurses while monitoring the patients. It contains therefore information on the response of the patient to the treatment and on the health status of a patient. It is written in a relatively subjective manner in comparison to other clinical narratives. Acronyms and typos appear very often in nurse letters due to the time pressure in the daily work of nurses.

A radiological report is mainly used to inform the treating physician about the findings of a radiological examination. It starts usually with an anamnesis, which is followed by a description of the region of interest and of observations on the inspected items. The text contains judgements and observations made during the examination. Finally, a discharge summary includes all the important aspects of a hospital stay of a patient. It starts normally with the patient information and medical history, which is followed by the diagnosis and applied medical interventions. Prescribed drugs, conclusion of the treatment process as well as suggestions for the further treatment constitute the last part of the summary.

An additional dataset comprises 24 surgical reports collected from RiteCode Website [45]. They cover different surgical fields (e.g. mammoplasty, sterilization, nasal surgery). The texts were originally provided as coding exercise. They are structured into paragraphs. The beginning of each paragraph is marked by headings such as "Diagnosis", "Name of operation", "Anesthesia", "Procedure". Sometimes, these headings are written in capital letters.

Different methods have been developed or applied to gain the information introduced in this book:

- Qualitative research for studying peculiarities of medical social media data,
- Literature review for collecting state of the art in ethical issues,
- Technical design and implementation using machine learning technology, adaptation of algorithms, selection of relevant features.

---

[1]http://www.physionet.org/.

Table 3.2 Datasets exploited in the book

Name	Size	Description	Source
Clinical documents	1000 per type	Nurse letters, discharge summaries, radiological reports	http://www.physionet.org/
MSM dataset	12,800 texts	Patient- and physician-written blog postings, two thirds of the collected blogs are provided by health professionals.	65 blogs from multiple sources
Drug reviews	1000 texts	Reviews on medications provided by laymen	http://www.drugratingz.com
Interview	1000 texts	Technical interviews	http://slashdot.org
Surgical reports	24 texts	Surgical reports provided as coding exercise	http://www.ritecode.com/

All data material is in English

Part II
Medical Social Media: Content, Characteristics, Appearance

Tweets, blog postings, forum entries—we can find a manifold landscape of medical content and social media tools in the web. This part provides an overview on available medical social media data and tools used for communicating medical information. Given the informal nature of communication, it is clear that language and content differs from other medical text types. The differences will be identified through a comparison of language characteristics in medical social media data and clinical documents.

Chapter 4
Types of Medical Social Media

There is a large variety of social media types available and in use in the context of healthcare and medicine. They can be broadly placed into two categories. Users can either generate their own content, or alternatively annotate the content created by others. To make the distinction clear, we refer to the former as **(user-generated) content**, and the latter as **metadata** (see Table 4.1).

Consider the following examples: in a weblog an individual person is providing content, (e.g. a person describes his experiences in living with a disease in his blog). In a wiki, content is produced collaboratively by multiple persons. In review and rating portals, opinions and experiences are assigned to drugs, health providers etc., i.e. metadata is generated.

Even though this book focuses on textual social media, for demonstrating the broad range of content and tools, in the following, examples of medical social media are described in more detail that are textual or non-textual. *Medical Video-Blogs (VLog)* provide information on medical issues in an audio-visual manner. A huge source of videos is available within the YouTube portal (e.g. the channel of the Mayo Clinic [10] or NHS choices [46]). The variety of videos ranges from recorded surgeries, educational videos for patients or medical students, to reports on medical issues in news channels. Authors of VLogs are health professionals, official health institutions and organizations, or universities. However, less professional content is also provided by non-health professionals.

Medical podcasts provide audio data with medical information. Podcasts offered by physicians inform patients about concrete health questions. Patient information on treatments (e.g. endoscopy, coronary angiography) or explanations of symptoms or diseases (e.g. obstructive sleep apnoea) are provided through podcasts of official organizations such as the Mayo Clinic [47]. Podcasts directed to physicians help to inform them about general issues or latest news such as medical informatics or electronic prescription. In addition, podcasts and video lectures are available for medical education purposes.

© Springer International Publishing Switzerland 2015
K. Denecke, *Health Web Science*, Health Information Science,
DOI 10.1007/978-3-319-20582-3_4

Table 4.1 Categories of medical social media data

	Collaborative	Non-collaborative
Content	Medical wiki	Blog, micro-blog, video-blog, podcasts, personal health records
Metadata	Social bookmarking, social networks	Review and rating portals, question and answer portals

Forums and query-answer portals (e.g. the forum DiabetesDaily [48]) with a medical focus offer the opportunity to post queries or engage in discussions. Expert forums enable patients or their relatives to get a qualified answer to a question regarding a disease or treatment. In such portals, patients' objective of posting is mainly to receive information related to drugs and disorders, with some attention also given to treatment-related issues [49]. Depending on the portal, answers can be provided either by health professionals or by the general public.

Content communities and social networking sites with health-related content enable people with similar interests to connect. More specifically, patients who suffer from diseases can share health data in order to empathise with each other or learn about treatments, physical exercises or medications other sufferers are consuming in order to improve their health status. Health professionals exploit social networking sites to connect with other professionals who share common (medical) interests. Yet other social networking sites such as HelloHealth [50] connect patients to physicians. PatientsLikeMe [51] is a social network for patients that allows to share health-related experiences and compare treatments. The community currently comprises more than 250,000 patient members (April, 2014). Over 2000 conditions are reported in the platform.

Weblogs or blogs are similar to paper-based diaries, that are normally kept by individuals and shared with others. Similar to a paper-based diary, the authors describe their personal opinions, impressions, feelings. As we will see later in this part of the book, patients are using blogs to describe their experiences with treatments, with living with a disease etc. Blog entries can be commented by others, which can lead to discussions within a blog.

In *review portals* users can anonymously rate the quality of medical products or even of healthcare providers. In drug reviews, for example, patients rate a drug with respect to several criteria, including effectiveness, side effects, convenience and value. They can also post comments, and see the public comments posted by others. The comments describe symptoms and side effects that occurred while taking a specific drug, or whether the medication was helpful or not. Similarly, doctors or other healthcare provider can be rated in corresponding rating portals (e.g. RateMD [52]).

Wikis provide a knowledge source where content is often collaboratively produced. For example, physician-written wikis focus on diseases, anatomy, drugs and medical procedures (e.g. surgeries) [49]. Target audience are often students of medicine or physicians. Collaborative writing targets at collecting and critically

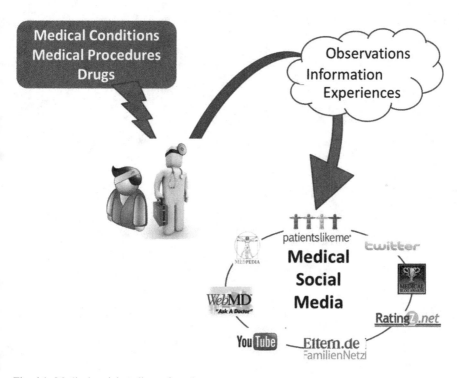

Fig. 4.1 Medical social media: tools and content

appraising the literature or at promoting the dissemination and application of the best available evidence to medical treatment (Fig. 4.1).

To summarise, the medical social web comprises content and metadata which is either generated collaboratively or non-collaboratively. Depending on the type, medical social media tools allow to

- Exchange information on diseases or treatments (e.g. forums, chats, podcasts, VLogs),
- Post information items such as images, messages, videos,
- Form groups (e.g. in social networks), or
- Work collaboratively on content (e.g. in wikis).

Chapter 5
Excursus: Content and Language in Clinical Narratives

This chapter provides a brief overview on the content and language peculiarities of clinical documents to have a reference for a comparison to content and language in medical blogs and medical social media.

5.1 Content of Clinical Documents

Medical data occurs in different data types: narrative, textual data, numerical measurements (e.g. vital signs), recorded signals (e.g. ECG) or pictures (e.g. radiologic images). It can comprise morphological, functional data, static or dynamic data. A medical datum is considered a single observation on a patient. It is defined by four elements:

- Patient in question,
- Parameter being observed,
- Value of the parameter in question, and
- Time of the observation.

A few examples of clinical data are listed in Table 5.1. In clinical documents, such data is described. They serve as documentation of the clinical assessments and as summary of the treatment. They mainly reflect the observations of physicians and health carers and are required for legal or billing issues or for communication purposes (e.g. for information exchange between physicians). They contain information on diagnosis, medications, complications occurred during a treatment, on findings etc. Beyond, biochemical information (e.g. gas exchange in the lungs), functional information (e.g. blood flow in vessels) or morphological information (e.g. CT scan) is often part of clinical data.

K. Denecke, *Health Web Science*, Health Information Science, DOI 10.1007/978-3-319-20582-3_5

Table 5.1 Examples for clinical data

Data type	Examples
Biochemical information	Gas exchange in lung
	Clearance of kidney
Functional information	Flow in blood vessels
	Elastomechanics of bone and soft tissue, contraction of muscle and tension development in skeletal muscle, metabolism in tumour
	PET scan
Morphological information	CT scan (static)
	Ultrasound of heart (dynamic)
	Electromyographic signals
Clinical findings	Diagnoses
	Symptoms
Medical procedures	Surgical intervention
	Radiotherapy
Information on quality of life	Physical and mental illness
	Self-perceived health
	Productivity
	Healthy behaviours
Experiences and observations	Drug consumption
	Perceptions of effectiveness of treatments
	Personal symptom perception

Several types of clinical documents can be distinguished: an *imaging report* describes what can be seen in a radiological image, the corresponding finding and its interpretation. The radiologist formulates in his own words the observations and interpretations. In contrast, *laboratory reports* are often structured and include the measured values or point out whether something was found or not. A *discharge summary* is a free textual description written at the end of a treatment process and summarises the hospital stay of a patient (which procedures were taken, which diagnoses have been assured, which medications have been prescribed). It can be structured into sections including anamnesis, finding, diagnosis, progress, medical procedures and type of discharge. *Pathology reports* document findings of histological assessments, i.e. of a microscopic analysis of some tissue or of some surgical preparation. They document a malignant tissue was recognized and provide information on the analysis methods, interpretation, or special tissue properties. *Operation records* describe the suite of actions during an operation and summarize the observations made during a surgery.

In summary, clinical narratives describe normally the health status of a person, observations, diagnoses and procedures in an objective manner. Personal impressions expressed in clinical documents concern perceptions of a health carer towards a patient's health status (e.g. the phrase *patient recovered well*) and interpretations of medical images and data.

5.2 The Sublanguage in Clinical Narratives

To study the peculiarities of the medical social media language in comparison to clinical documents, we will apply methods similar to sublanguage analysis. In the 1990s, Zellig Harris [53] introduced sublanguage theory, a theory of information content. Zellig claimed that languages of technical domains have a certain structure and regularity which can be specified in computer-processable manner. In contrast to the general grammar theory, Harris's sublanguage theory incorporates domain-specific semantic information and syntactic peculiarities of a domain language. Thus, a sublanguage is the language of a restricted domain, for example the medical domain, and in this way a subset of a natural language characterized by the fact that only a subset of the vocabulary and certain grammatical rules are used. From this theory, sublanguage analysis has been applied to study language patterns and peculiarities. Sublanguage analysis is a technique for discovering units of information and their relationships in narrative text.

According to Friedman [54] the following characteristics are relevant within such analysis:

- Semantic categorization of terms,
- Co-occurrence patterns or constraints,
- Context-specific omission of information,
- Usage of terminologies and controlled vocabularies,
- Mix of sublanguage-specific and general language patterns.

The clinical sublanguage was comprehensively analysed within the context of developing natural language processing tools for clinical documents and compared to the biomedical sublanguage [54], to general English [55] and to newspaper language. Sager and Nhan described the sublanguage in clinical documents together with implications for its automatic processing [56]. Following these results, the clinical sublanguage is characterized by compact formulations, resisting on verbs and extensive use of nouns and compound words. The documents contain many expressions with numbers and measurements. Given the mixture of languages (Latin, Greek, and the host language), there are multiple spellings of words as well as synonyms (e.g. typhlitis, appendicitis) available to a large extent. Abbreviations are frequently used and created on the fly.

One of the most often used mean to analyse the (clinical) sublanguage, is a study of word usage. Friedman et al. determined semantic categories of words, and co-occurrence patterns of words and semantic categories to study and compare clinical and biomedical sublanguage [54]. They found out that the clinical sublanguage is characterised by a usage of words belonging to the semantic categories *Behaviour, Findings, Medication, Device, Bodyfunction, Labtest, Procedure* [54]. Additionally, there are modifiers used in the texts, i.e. words that are only meaningful when they modify other concepts or relations. Modifiers in clinical documents fall among others into the categories *Bodylocation, Certainty or Degree* (e.g. *left arm, no evidence, very severe*). In Sect. 6.2, we will compare the social media sublanguage to the sublanguage in clinical documents by means of a study of word usage.

Chapter 6
Content and Language in Medical Social Media

Medical social-media data are written for other purposes than clinical texts and biomedical literature, even though authors can be healthcare professionals, clinical researchers as well as non-health professionals. Thus, the literary style of medical social media data is markedly different. Whereas the linguistic characteristics of clinical and biomedical texts have been analysed in painstaking detail by other researchers [54, 57, 58] (see Sect. 5.2), the literary composition of medical social media data has not yet been analysed with the same degree of precision. Being aware of the linguistic peculiarities of that particular data is crucial when developing tools for language processing and data analysis. In this section, we will have a closer look at the characteristics of the language of medical social media data as well as to the content in comparison to clinical narratives.

6.1 Content of Medical Blogs

The content and language of a medical social media text can be influenced by the author, his intention and by the social media type used (e.g. blogs, microblog). The intent or "mission" of an author is often either sharing experiences or distributing medical knowledge. Consider the following example: A person suffering from diabetes describes in her blog her daily experience with living with diabetes. Her main interest is in sharing her experiences. From time to time, she provides information on treatments she became aware of. Texts are characterized by personal experiences, contain facts, but also opinions, feelings etc. In contrast, a physician specialised in diabetes treatment intends to inform his patients on treatment options, on the importance of blood sugar measurement and on other issues related to diabetes treatment. His language is more official due to his intent to inform people and to provide evidence-based information.

© Springer International Publishing Switzerland 2015   33
K. Denecke, *Health Web Science*, Health Information Science,
DOI 10.1007/978-3-319-20582-3_6

Further, the social media type or tool that is used for distributing the information influences the language. As described before, multiple social media tools exist, and they have each a different audience. Considering the social media type, it is clear that *microblogs* contain only limited information given the restriction of a maximum of 160 characters per message. Many abbreviations are exploited to communicate sufficient information despite the limited message length. In *forums and question/answer portals*, the spectrum in content comprises short questions up to complete histories of illness. Answers can be either short or comprehensive. In the following, we are concentrating on content of medical blogs as an example for medical social media data.

Blogs are comprehensive texts. They can provide many details and are often also enriched with hyperlinks, images etc. Since a blog is a kind of personal diary, it is not surprising that personal opinions are often freely expressed. To get insights into the content of medical blogs, we will have a closer look to four different blogs of the data set. More specifically, posts from two patient-written blogs (Stellarlife, Blog from Randy Pausch) and from two physician-written blogs (WebMD, KevinMD) were manually analysed addressing the questions:

- How often new postings are provided?
- What is the content and focus of writing?
- Which specific medical content is described?

A sample of blog postings of these sources were randomly selected and analysed to answer these questions. The posts of Stellarlife [37] are written by a woman suffering from multiple sclerosis. The blog starts in 2007 and the author is still active with around three to four posts per month. The blog includes the author's views on current events, disability issues, politics, and health issues. When writing about her personal health, she focuses on treatments and medications. The blog provides insights into the difficulties in living with multiple sclerosis.

In contrast, the blog from Randy Pausch [38] (former professor of computer science at Carnegie Mellon University) presents clinical data and laboratory results such as blood marker, radiological images, or weight. Between 2006 and 2008, new postings were added by Pausch or his wife five to ten times per months, before he died from cancer. This blog provides objectively clinical values, and the symptoms and side effects of the treatment he is undergoing are described. The progress of the disease becomes visible in all its facets, changes or problems of the health status, dealing with family issues and job etc. Beyond, some general statistics of the treatment options were given and the radiological images were described in a lay man language.

Interestingly, the physician-written blogs stay general, almost not describing patient cases. In blogs hosted by WebMD [40], physicians write about topics related to health and medicine. The main focus in the analysed postings was on treatment. Authors give advice and explain symptoms (e.g. vomiting in children and when to go to the doctor). Beside this, they are providing personal experiences regarding nutrition and wellness, reflect about journal articles, or new treatments. New postings are added several times a month.

Since its start in 2004, KevinMD [9] becomes a prominent social media platform with over one million monthly page views and is regularly cited by the Wall Street Journal, New York Times, USA Today, and CNN. Over 1000 authors contribute to KevinMD.com: front-line primary care doctors, surgeons, specialist physicians, nurses, medical students, policy experts, and patients. Authors of postings provide information on medical treatments, or clinical decision making, on health topics or interpret spectacular patient cases that were presented in the press. Additionally, the patient-doctor relationship is reflected.

Even this small assessment shows that patients rather describe in blog postings their experiences in living with a disease and in receiving some medical treatment. In contrast, physicians try to inform by providing details on treatments. Compared to clinical documents, blog content is rather experiential. However, clinical data including laboratory results or radiological images are sometimes posted also through social media channels. They are extended by personal observations and measurements from patients. The main content overlap between medical blogs and clinical narratives are mentions of symptoms, disorders and medical treatments, medications (see Fig. 6.1). Morphological or biochemical information is normally not included in private blogs. On the other hand, lifestyle information and personal observations of patients are not described in clinical documents.

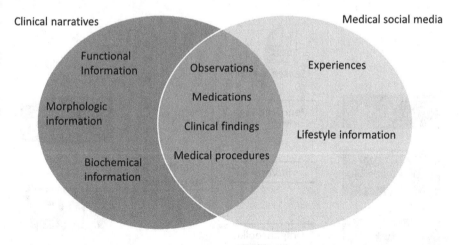

Fig. 6.1 Medical social media and clinical data: content overlap can be found in mentions of medications, clinical findings, medical procedures and observations

6.2   Word Usage in Medical Social Media: A Linguistic Analysis

6.2.1   Sublanguage Analysis of Medical Social Media

To study the characteristics of the medical social media sublanguage, we determined linguistic and semantic patterns. More specifically, we studied verb usage, semantic categories of words, and co-occurrence patterns of semantic categories with verbs. The objective was to identify similarities and differences between the language in clinical documents and in medical social media and to draw conclusions for developing tools for automatic processing of medical social media data.

The following tools and methods were applied to a data set of medical blogs to study the language and content patterns:

- Part of speech tagging with Penn Tree POS-tagger [59],
- Relation extraction with ReVerb,
- Mapping to concepts of the UMLS Metathesaurus with DragonToolkit,
- Lexicon lookup with subjectivity lexicon [60] and SentiWordNet.

For comparison, we apply the same methods also to a set of clinical documents and non-medical social media. The analysis process is depicted in Fig. 6.2. We chose the open information extraction tool ReVerb [61] for extracting relations in form of two arguments connected by a relation type without the need of specifying relation

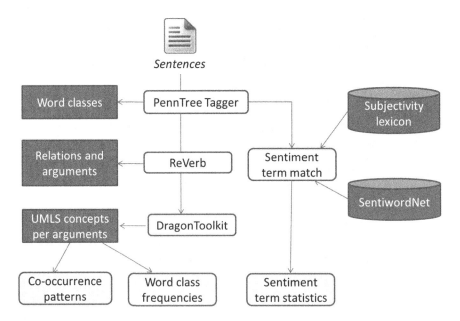

Fig. 6.2 Processing steps for the sublanguage analysis

types of interest. ReVerb is designed for web-scale information extraction, where the target relations cannot be specified in advance and speed is important [61]. To determine parts of speech of words, we applied the Penn Tree POS-tagger. For identifying medical concepts, the biomedical text annotator MaxMatcher provided within the DragonToolkit [62] was exploited. It uses a generic extraction approach (referred to as "approximate dictionary lookup") to cope with term variations. A precision rate of 71.6 % and a recall of 75 % was achieved [62] on biomedical abstracts collected from MEDLINE. DragonToolkit was not yet evaluated on medical social media data. The underlying terminology of MaxMatcher is the Unified Medical Language System (UMLS) (version UMLS 2004AA Version). Details on the UMLS are provided in Sect. 8.2.2.

Co-occurrence patterns as collected in our sublanguage analysis consist of one or two sets of UMLS main categories and a verb. They are received by applying ReVerb to a sentence. The left and right argument extracted by ReVerb are processed by the DragonToolkit to map text to UMLS concepts and to get semantic categories of the words in the argument string. An example of a co-occurrence pattern is: *[Procedures + show + Disorders]* (e.g. the sentence *Head CT from the outside hospital showed blood in the basal cisterns.*). The left argument is mapped to a concept of the semantic category *Procedures* and the right argument to a concept of the semantic category *Disorders*. The two sentiment lexicons, Subjectivity Lexicon [60] (SL, contains 8221 single-term subjective expressions) and SentiWordNet (SWN, contains 117,659 single terms), have been used to study the use of opinionated terms in the data set. We applied an exact matching algorithm.

The data set underlying our study comprises 1000 randomly selected texts from the MSM data set (referred to as "MedBlog" in this chapter), drug reviews, slashdot dataset and clinical documents. The clinical documents consist of each 1000 nurse letters, discharge summaries and radiology reports. More details on these data sets are described in Sect. 3.3.

Within a **quantitative comparison**, we analysed and compared the word usage of the six text types. The MedBlogs, Slashdot interviews and the drug reviews are typical user generated content. We expect that these three corpora will contain a large amount of sentiment terms and subjective expressions, while the clinical narratives are expected to be written in a more objective way. Less opinionated terms and more clinical terminology are expected. However, the question is whether the terminology and word usage is really distributed as expected. To what extent do the corpora differ with respect to linguistic characteristics? In the following sections, results of the sublanguage analysis are described.

6.2.2   Statistics of Word Classes

In Fig. 6.3, for each text source the proportions of nouns, adjectives, verbs, adverbs and stop words are illustrated. Figure 6.4 presents the percentage of extracted sentiment terms. Apparently, the six text sources are different in terms of terminology usage and content. A more detailed discussion per word class follows.

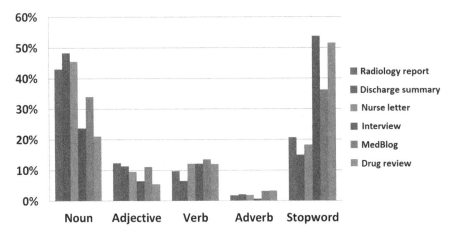

Fig. 6.3 Quantitative assessment of parts of speech in the six corpora

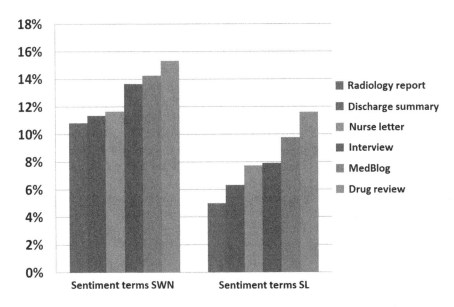

Fig. 6.4 Quantitative assessment of sentiment terms in the six corpora ("SWN - SentiWordNet; SL - Subjectivity lexicon")

Nouns

Compared to the other word classes, nouns are the most frequently used parts of speech in all datasets. What noteworthy is, the percentage of nouns in clinical documents (e.g., radiology reports (42.9 %), and clinical documents (48 %)) is clearly higher than the percentage of nouns in the other text sources (e.g. in interviews (23.7 %) or drug reviews (21 %)). The reason is that medical facts are described in clinical narratives in a very compact manner, in a so-called nominal style (e.g. names of diseases, symptoms, medications, treatments are listed). They are summarizing facts, while the other document types are rather observational, describing observations and judgements. In drug reviews, the number of nouns is particularly low. This is due to the fact that in these reviews mainly impressions and feelings with respect to drug efficacy are expressed. Interestingly, the number of nouns in the MedBlog data set is also quite high (34 %) compared to the other social media data sets.

Adjectives

Another interesting finding is that the clinical narratives and texts from medical blogs contain a substantial amount of adjectives (9–12 % of the terms). In contrast, adjectives occur less frequently in the interview corpus and in drug reviews. Through manual inspection, we recognized that the adjectives used in the clinical narratives are mainly related to body locations, such as "left" side, "right" side, "vertical", "dorsal", "cervical". They express neither emotion nor attitude, but anatomical concepts and relative locations in the body. The MedBlog dataset contains a similar amount of adjectives, which is also due to the description of body locations in the texts.

Stop Words

Interestingly, the number of stop words is very large for the social media data sets with 51 % in the drug reviews, 36 % in the MedBlogs and even 53 % in the interview data set. In contrast, the nurse letters, radiology reports and discharge summaries contain 18, 20 and 14 % stop words, respectively. This demonstrates that the clinical documents are clearly written in a much more concise way, focussing on facts and resisting on using meaningless words.

Verbs

With respect to verbs, we can recognize that except for clinical documents, between 10 and 14 % of the terms are verbs. In clinical documents, significantly less verbs could be identified. This again reflects the fact that these documents are written in a more nominal style, listing facts, while the other text types report also actions and behaviours. The number of adverbs is very low for all datasets. Verbs that are used frequently in medical social media texts fall into the following categories:

- **Verbs describing effects of medical procedures, drugs and proteins or genes:** affect, regulate, reduce, prevent, improve, help, treat, increase, enhance, enable, benefit, strengthen,
- **Verbs describing observations:** appear,
- **Verbs referring to education and research** learn, discuss, study, empower, educate,
- **Verbs describing disease development and transfer:** contribute, depend, infect, require, acquire,

Note that verb forms of *be, have* and *do* were not considered even though they had a high frequency as well. In contrast, frequently used verbs in discharge documents mainly fall into two categories: they are referring to **administrative issues of patient treatment** (e.g., *admit, discharge, transfer, continue*) or **describing observations** (e.g., *show, reveal, present, demonstrate, tolerate*).

6.2.3   Sentiment Terms

The analysis of term matches with the two sentiment lexicons (SL, SWN) shows similar trends for both lexicons [63] (see Fig. 6.4): The drug reviews contain the highest proportion of sentiment terms with 11.6 % (SL) and 15.3 % (SWN), followed by the MedBlog with 9.7 % (SL) and 14.2 % (SWN) (Table 6.1). In contrast, much less words in the radiology reports and in the clinical documents match the SL and SWN. This confirms the more subjective language in social media data sets. Even between the different types of clinical narratives, we can recognize differences: Nurse letters contain more opinionated terms than the other two clinical datasets. They are written in a more subjective manner than radiology reports, but they are still more objective than the social media texts. This result confirms our initial hypothesis that nurse letters are more subjectively written than other clinical narratives.

Table 6.1 Percentage of sentiment terms (positive and negative) extracted from the six sources using SL and SWN

Sources	Subjectivity lexicon			SentiWordNet		
	Positive (%)	Negative (%)	Total (%)	Positive (%)	Negative (%)	Total (%)
Radiology report	61	39	5	46	53	10.8
Nurse letter	58	42	8	51	49	11.6
Discharge summary	52	48	6	48	52	11.3
Interview	52	48	8	56	44	13
Drug review	48	52	12	46	54	15.3
MedBlog	51	49	10	56	43	14

After manually reviewing the text material, we could recognize that the sentiments expressed in nurse letters are normally implicit and appear together with the
description of patient's health status, or the social records for the visitors of the
patients. Opinionated terms and expressions such as suspicion, negation, approval
or recommendations can be found in radiology reports mainly in the conclusion
section or impression part at the end of the whole report. In contrast, sentiment
terms are distributed over the complete text in the social media data sets.

Another interesting result is that the two lexicons obviously have a different
coverage. Much more sentiment terms were identified by applying SWN. To inves-
tigate the identified sentiment terms, we determined the proportion of adjectives and
nouns that were extracted as sentiment terms through application of both lexicons.
Second, we identified the top 10 frequent terms per lexicon and corpus to judge their
concrete content.

Through these statistics we learned that matches with SentiWordNet occur
frequently with nouns: Around 17–47 % of the sentiment term matches with SWN
are nouns. In contrast, only 7–14 % of the matches with SL are nouns. The top
frequent terms confirmed again that SWN already covers a certain amount of
medical terms which is in contrast to the SL result. For instance, in the radiology
reports, nouns such as "pneumothorax", "artery" have been recognized as sentiment
terms using SWN. Frequent terms extracted using the SL were adjectives such as
"significant" or "well". In addition, frequent matches with SWN were adjectives
describing anatomical locations such as "bilateral", "upper","subclavian" "inferior".
The analysis using the SL did not recognized these terms. We conclude that SWN
matches more terms in the medical documents. However, the matching results also
contain many objective terms. This is in contrast to matches recognized using the
SL, where only subjective terms are included and therefore extracted. Moreover, the
top frequency term statistics has also indicated that the polarity of certain adjectives
needs to be adapted before an application to clinical documents. For example, the
terms "patient" or "normal" have a different polarity in SWN than it is expected in
medical documents.

6.2.4   Semantic Categories

Content differences become clear when looking at the top three main categories
of extracted concepts. In clinical documents, words mainly belong frequently to
the semantic categories *Procedures, Disorders, Anatomy, Concepts and Ideas*.
In contrast, words identified in medical social media data belong often to the
category *Living Beings*. In addition, words falling into the categories *Disorders,
Chemicals and Drugs, Concept and Ideas* are exploited frequently.

It becomes clear that the focus in clinical documents is on *procedures, disorders,
symptoms* and *anatomy* while authors of blogs frequently use terms referring to
disorders and *living beings*. The UMLS category *Concept and Ideas* contains rather
unspecific words such as temporal terms (e.g. *six to eight weeks*) or quantitative
terms (e.g. *severe*) and are extracted from all data sets frequently. Words falling into

the category *Chemical and Drugs* are in position four for clinical documents, so also quite often used. Medical procedures do not occur very frequently in medical blogs. In contrast, clinical documents describe the medical procedures performed during the hospital stay of a patient reflected by a frequent use of concepts representing medical procedures.

Words falling into the category *Living Being* are extracted for example from the following sentences of the blog data set: *According to the CDC, in 2006 (the latest data available) an estimated 106,374* **men** *and 90,080* **women** *were diagnosed in the U.S. with lung cancer.*, or the sentence *Within days of having a tiny microchip surgically implanted, the two* **men** *and one* **woman** *could see shadows and were able to recognise some shapes.* It can be seen that general statistical information is provided instead of referring to an individual. This is clearly in contrast to clinical documents, where the focus is on one concrete patient. In the latter, reference to the patient is normally made by personal pronouns (e.g. *he, she*) which are not identified by the methods applied in our analysis. Thus, they are not detected as references to concepts of type *Living Beings* and thus do not occur frequently in clinical documents. Table 6.2 lists for both data sets, clinical documents and medical blogs, frequently used verbs, main categories and semantic types.

6.2.5   Semantic Patterns

The pattern analysis was performed for clinical documents in comparison to medical blogs and resulted in frequently used co-occurrence patterns. They are listed in Table 6.3. Patterns that occur in both data sets frequently are referring to having or developing diseases or symptoms and performing actions/medical procedures

Table 6.2 Frequent main groups, semantic types and verbs for clinical documents and medical blogs

Text type	Top 3 main categories	Top 5 semantic types	Top 10 verbs
Clinical documents	Procedures, Disorders, Anatomy, Concepts and ideas	[Disease or syndrome], [Therapeutic or preventive procedure], [Finding], [Body part, Organ, or organ component], [Diagnostic procedure]	Show, reveal, admit, discharge, receive, transfer, present, demonstrate, tolerate, continue
Medical blogs	Living beings, Disorders, Chemicals and drugs, Concept and ideas	[Disease or syndrome], [Finding], [Family group], [Therapeutic or preventive procedure], [Quantitative concept]	Say, include, get, take, make, cause, found, affect, increase, publish, improve, visit, develop, require, appear

Table 6.3 Frequent co-occurrence patterns in clinical documents and medical blogs

Clinical documents	Medical blogs
• **Patterns referring to diagnosed diseases** (e.g., *[have + Disorders]*, *[develop + Disorders]*) • **Patterns referring to performed actions** (e.g., *[Procedures + show + Disorders]*, *[Procedures + be]*, *[Procedures + reveal + Disorders]*) and • **Patterns referring to general administration information** (e.g. *[admit + Organizations]*)	• **Patterns referring to having or developing diseases or symptoms** (e.g. *[have + Disorders]*, *[develop + Disorders]*), • **Patterns on drug consumption** (e.g., *[take + Chemicals and Drugs]*, *[receiv + Chemicals and Drugs]*), • **Patterns representing statements of persons on medical issues** (e.g. *[Living Beings + say + Concepts and Ideas, Phenomena]*, *[say + Living Beings]*, and • **Patterns referring to the use of devices for confirming a diagnosis or performing procedures** (e.g. *[Devices + discov + Disorders, Procedures]*).

A pattern consists of a verb and one or two sets of main groups, here separated by a "+"

including drug consumption. A pattern referring to hospital administrative tasks is occurring only in clinical documents frequently, which is clearly related to the content of these documents.

Additionally, in medical social media texts patterns occur frequently that are used to describe the use of medical devices and those representing statements of persons on medical issues. Even though there is some overlap in patterns, it becomes clear that the content in blogs is broader, provides more variety than clinical documents.

6.2.6 Additional Characteristics of Blogs

In addition to the results from the sublanguage analysis, we are summarizing some additional observations made while manually reading blog postings of the data set. Blogs can refer to an individual person, but contain seldom measured values. In our blog data set, authors often refer to general health statistics or health information in their texts.

Personal pronouns are exploited frequently (e.g., *I saw, I experienced* or *My daughter is sick*). Furthermore, **rather long sentences** are prevalent, containing a **wealth of adjectives** to describe situations, experiences, impressions, etc. Postings are written in common everyday language—even using language that is modern and hip—so as to appeal to the average reader. An example from the multiple sclerosis blog Stellarlife illustrates this point: "Yesterday I finally got to see an orthopedic, okay hold the buggy, I just googled the guy and he is a PA-C/MPAS!! Shut the front door! That means: Physician's Assistant-Certified/Masters Physician's Assistant Studies—huh."

While the intent is to use **everyday language**, the insertion of medical terminology in a posting, be it a blog, actually depends entirely on the content of each posting. For example, when a person is writing about their experiences with a disease, the corresponding terminology is used, sometimes even with explanations of the clinical terms. Here is a snippet from the blog Diabetesmine to illustrate this pattern: "No one is sure what causes this dead-in-bed syndrome, but the theory is that a nighttime low blood sugar—called a nocturnal low—episode triggers some kind of fatal cardiac arrhythmia."

Another distinction between social media postings and clinical texts is that in the former, **abbreviations are often explained** in the text of the posting itself. In addition, sometimes words or word phrases are typographically highlighted. This can be done via the use of full caps, quotation marks around a word or word phrase, or other stylistic means of allowing parts of the text to stand out more saliently. We draw again from the blog Diabetesmine to make this point: *While many parents are likely relieved to "get a break" and have their kids back in class, this can be a very stressful experience for the parents of Children With Diabetes (CWDs) who have a LOT more to worry about than just textbooks and extracurricular activities.* In this sentence, the word "lot" was highlighted by using capital letters.

Repetition of information or statements from another person, often a high profile scientist or public official who has something to say about a major health issue, is another phenomenon in medical social media. In Diabetesmine, we found that the blogger inserted a quote from a high profile scientist to support her own contention about the danger of sugar levels dropping precipitously at night: "We've now known for decades that (overnight) is the most common time for severe hypoglycemia," says Dr. Irl Hirsch, assistant professor and endocrinologist at the University of Washington, and a type 1 PWD himself.". From this example sentence, we can also recognize that in blog postings, **named entities occur such as person names, organization names or locations**.

Not only do blogs contain certain kinds of conversational features, as illustrated above, they are also very much prone to short block paragraphs and bullet point itemization. Bloggers have been found likewise to give headings to their postings as a way of categorising the content of their blogs. However, these headings are not fix as they are in clinical documents where sections often start with standardized headings such as *Anamnesis* or *Diagnoses*.

6.3 Implications for Automatic Processing

The characteristics presented before demonstrated many differences between the language and content in blogs or medical social media, respectively, and clinical documents which is certainly due to the different purposes of the documents. In summary, language in medical social media has the following characteristics:

- Mixture of facts and experiences or opinions,
- Frequent use of personal pronouns and verbs,
- Variety of adjectives,
- Use of everyday language combined with medical terminology,

Table 6.4 Linguistic characteristics of clinical texts, and medical social media texts, here specifically blogs

Text type	Clinical text	Medical social media
Sentence structure	Ungrammatical sentences; short, telegraphic phrases (e.g. *Aspirin or Fever*); often without verbs or other relational operators	Rather long sentences
Word usage	Word compounds (*high blood pressure*), formed ad hoc; modifiers are related to temporal information (e.g. sudden), evidential information (e.g. rule out, no evidence), severity information (mild, extensive), body location	Adjectives; descriptive and narrative words
Spelling	Misspellings; abbreviations, acronyms	Abbreviations, misspellings
Language	Mix of Latin and Greek roots with corresponding host language (German, English); domain-specific language	Common language, rather than domain-specific language or clinical terminology; host language
Semantic categories of words	Procedures, disorders, anatomy, concepts and ideas	Living beings, disorders, chemicals and drugs, concept and ideas

- Use of abbreviations or acronyms together with their explanations,
- Repetition of information or statements made by others and
- Use of named entities including person names, locations and organizations.

Table 6.4 summarises the linguistic characteristics of clinical texts and textual medical social media.

At present, the existing text-mining tools have been specifically developed for processing clinical and biomedical texts, whose language usage and content differs significantly from medical social media as the sublanguage analysis showed. The differing sublanguage of medical social media texts still poses several challenges for automatic processing tools.

Verbs are used in free text to generate relations between concepts, e.g. between disease names and procedures, causes and symptoms etc. which is important information to be identified during an automatic analysis. The broader spectrum of verbs used in medical blogs results in a need for **tools that are able to collect these verbs and analyse their meanings** when it comes to automatic interpretation of social media text. The variety in verbs exploited in medical social media texts makes it difficult to specify in advance verb patterns or extraction rules that contain verbs. Since, the clinical sublanguage often resists on verbs, the existing text analysis tools for the clinical domain do not process verbs and their meanings.

Given the fact that in social media many references to living beings are made, it is crucial to have **methods on hand for identifying the referred subject** and distinguishing it from the reporting person. It is important to identify what is said about whom and what. In clinical documents, it is clear, that all diagnoses and procedures mentioned refer to one patient. A challenge for automatic processing of medical social media texts that contain verbatim quotes is that in order to have a correct reference to the quote, a processing algorithm must correctly link the cited person, and not the blog author, to the quote itself. Co-reference resolution algorithms are required for this task.

In medical social media, information provided can be general (e.g. general statistics of effectiveness of treatments) or specific (e.g. referring to a patient). Further, social media authors provide their personal experiences. These **different types of information need to be separated** correctly depending on the analysis objective or application behind. For example, when we want to build a system that analyses personal opinions expressed in social media texts written by physicians with respect to some treatment, general information described in the text need to be filtered out.

Additionally, tools for the automatic processing of medical social media need to consider a range of stylistic preferences in the presentation of the content, and the syntactic features characterising social media communications—which can be notoriously long-winded, ungrammatical, idiosyncratic as displayed by the use of full caps and italics for emphasis. In contrast to processing non-medical web content, the processing tools need to be able to capture the medical terminology and to identify described relations. In summary, entity recognition methods for identifying mentions of diseases, symptoms, procedures and medications as well as identifying common named entities such as person names, organisations and locations need to be available. Additional methods required include:

- Relation detection and verb interpretation methods,
- Reference detection methods,
- Co-reference resolution technologies,
- Classification methods for distinguishing facts from experiences and for analysing sentiment.

Given the more complex linguistic structures in medical social media, these technologies need to be available for adequately interpreting content in medical social media respectively. The challenges with respect to sentiment analysis are described in more detail in Chap. 10. Table 6.5 summarizes the language characteristics of medical social media texts and their implications for automatic processing.

Table 6.5 Implications of language and content characteristics of medical social media for automatic processing tools

Language characteristics of medical social media	Example	Implication for automatic processing
Abbreviations and named entities referring to organizations, persons, geographical locations	"CDC" (Center for Disease Prevention and Control)	Methods for named entity recognition and resolution of abbreviations
Medical abbreviations and their explanations	*This can be a very stressful experience for the parents of Children With Diabetes (CWDs)*	Methods for identification and resolution of abbreviations
Citations and statements from others	*"We've now known for decades that (overnight) is the most common time for severe hypoglycemia," says Dr. Irl Hirsch, assistant professor and endocrinologist at the University of Washington, and a type 1 PWD himself."*	Reference resolution methods
Personal pronouns	"he", "I"	Methods for resolution of pronoun references
Frequent use of verbs	*If I can continue my exercise routine, eat healthy, laugh, write, love and be loved, my years should be many.*	Relationship extraction methods, semantic mapping and analysis of verbs
Facts, attitudes, experiences	*I would take it again for my illness. It's potent and so far seems to be clearing up my lungs and sinuses!*	Methods for sentiment analysis, classification of subjective and objective texts, grouping along sentiments
Complex sentences	*It was 3AM and there I was trapped between my heavy power chair and the ceramic thrown. The poor carer pulled with all his might (I had the bruises to show it, in fact the knee scraping was due to his and the summoned medics trying to lift me up! The medics finally lifted my chair away and two of them got me seated back in my chair,) but I was stuck between too heavy devices.*	Relation extraction methods, reference resolution methods, semantic mapping and analysis of verbs, named entity recognition
Everyday language and medical terminology	*vomiting all day*	Availability of domain knowledge, medical terminology, consumer health vocabulary and corresponding extraction methods

Part III
Information Discovery from Medical Social Media

Many applications described in Chap. 2 that make use of written medical social media data, require an automatic analysis of these texts, e.g. for determining trends or health problems of a patient to generate automatic alerts. In this part, various methods will be introduced necessary to analyse and extract information from the data. We refer to applications that exploit social media data, analyse and process it for healthcare purposes with the general term *textanalytic-enabled applications*. A general architecture for such applications will be introduced. Extracting medical concepts from texts is a key issue in the context of information extraction from medical social media. We will see how existing tools for medical concept extraction perform on medical social media. Determining attitudes and opinions as well as distinguishing facts from experiences is another important issue. For this reason, the topic of sentiment analysis will be introduced and sentiment in the medical domain will be characterized since it differs from sentiment in other domains such as customer reviews. We will introduce relevant methods.

Chapter 7
Textanalytic-Enabled Healthcare Applications: Requirements and Architecture

Applications that analyse textual social media data for their exploitation in healthcare ("textanalytic-enabled systems") require methods for text analysis, visualisation, machine learning etc. Often, similar methods are used for different applications. Thus, a re-use of methods and components could facilitate the development of applications. In this chapter, we introduce a framework for developing textanalytic-enabled systems. After summarizing the requirements, the framework has to address, we describe the main components. In Chap. 11, it will be shown how the introduced architecture is implemented for developing a concrete application.

7.1 Textanalysis Tasks and Requirements

The requirements towards an architecture of a textanalytic-enabled system and its components can be grouped according to the various perspectives or actors of such system. The (a) end-user is working with a client application which enables access to the actual system. Normally, the end-user is not aware or caring about the underlying technology. The (b) system developer has the role to "plug" the different services together to create a new application addressing a concrete healthcare scenario. He does not necessarily have knowledge in text analysis or natural language processing (NLP), respectively or in implementing NLP components and services. The (c) service engineer creates and develops the processing services, for example NLP services for information extraction or named entity recognition. We resist on discussing the role of the service engineer here since our focus is on the general architecture of textanalytic-enabled applications, and not on the way how text analysis services or other services are implemented at the end. For system development, it should be of no concern how the components are created and which algorithms are exploited. In addition to the various user perspectives, we finally

© Springer International Publishing Switzerland 2015   51
K. Denecke, *Health Web Science*, Health Information Science,
DOI 10.1007/978-3-319-20582-3_7

assume the (d) system perspective, where we consider the properties desirable for the architecture as a whole. In the following sections, the various requirements are described in more detail.

7.1.1   End-User Requirements

In the medical domain, potential end users of textanalytic-enabled applications are doctors, nurses, patients or health carers. The activities and functions of these stakeholders can be structured into

- Treatment-centred activities,
- Knowledge management and gathering activities, and
- Research and monitoring activities

Treatment-centred activities focus on the patient and the treatment of his medical condition including direct interaction between healthcare provider and patient. These activities require access to clinical data, i.e. to examination results, documentations etc. Additionally, health carers and doctors need for example summaries of the information a patient has provided through social media tools and analytical tools that analyse changes in the health status as documented in social media texts to avoid additional work on physician side. Communication and data exchange among health carer and with patients should be enabled. Patients require tools for entering information on their health status using free text or supported by appropriate scales or visualisations. Therapists and physicians should be enabled to provide exercises or questionnaires to a patient. Replies from the patient need to be visualised and evaluated automatically. Relatives of patients only need to see status information. Means for interacting with the data and with other persons involved in the treatment process and methods to interact with the data through various visualisations is often necessary for all end-user groups (see Chap. 2).

Knowledge management and gathering activities concern activities where healthcare provider, or patients are gathering information from social media and web data such as information on diseases, treatment options or managing knowledge using social media tools. This requires search and retrieval facilities. In particular patients will exploit a different vocabulary for searching for information. They need support in formulating their information need in proper terms. Results need to be prepared in an user-friendly manner, e.g. as summaries, grouping of results according to topics.

Research and monitoring activities refer to all activities that are directed towards clinical research and public health. These activities require facilities to specify the symptoms or medical conditions under monitoring. Results need to be filtered, visualised and summarised appropriately.

Table 7.1 summarises activity types and resulting needs with respect to technology and information gathering. Taking into account the different user groups and scenarios, a textanalytic-enabled architecture must be open and flexible with respect

Table 7.1 End-user needs with respect to a textanalytic-enabled architecture grouped by activities

Activity	Information and technology needs
Treatment-centred activity	Data exchange and communication facilities; access to clinical data, guidelines, biomedical literature, and other clinical knowledge; facilities for entering data (providing descriptions of exercises, questionnaires, comments); visualizations for monitoring the health status
Knowledge management activities	Search and retrieval facilities for patient data, publications and other information; technologies for grouping and clustering of retrieval results; support in query formulation; information summarization methods
Research and monitoring activities	Methods for trend detection; support in specifying subjects of monitoring (symptoms or diseases)

to the type of clients integrated with. Further, methods for considering the user context and his role need to be implemented. Depending on the working context, a user might have different tasks and access rights. For instance, nurses can be able to check the current health status of a patient, but are not allowed to make any changes to clinical patient data. Since healthcare workflows might involve the use of various software applications, the architecture must allow for the automatic invocation of external applications such as connection to health information systems or to health monitoring systems (e.g. glucose monitoring system).

7.1.2 System Developer Requirements

System developers are a second user group. They create textanalytic-enabled applications that make use of social media data and integrate them into a client application. A component-based architecture aims at facilitating their job. For this reason, the architecture should allow for an easy integration of any client and should enable developers to do this in an effective and efficient manner. Further, reuse of components for analysis, processing and visualization is a main issue, since this may help to reduce the development effort significantly.

7.1.3 Architecture Requirements

Additional requirements are related to the architecture itself. Easy communication between client and server needs to be enabled. Considering the user requirements, processing services should support several tasks:

- **Collecting content:** Retrieve texts or other data from the web or other sources,
- **Filtering:** Select content relevant to address some task,
- **Extracting relevant information:** Extract symptoms mentioned by a patient in a forum, summarise the health status,

Table 7.2 Architecture requirements of a textanalytic-enabled systems

	Architecture requirements
1	Ensuring easy communication between client and server
2	Enabling easy modification, replacement and extension of knowledge resources
3	Enabling easy integration of new processing services
4	Enabling automatic invocation of external applications (e.g. enterprise-, desktop and web applications)
5	Ensure flexible handling of results
6	Methods for data analysis, collection, filtering and interpretation

- **Analysing and interpreting extracted information:** Summarise texts, determine trends or changes in the health status,
- **Visualising and interacting with information and data:** Show trends, enter data

Depending on the task addressed by a processing service, it requires different resources (e.g. lexicons, ontologies, data from databases). Easy maintenance of these sources, i.e. their easy modification, replacement or extension is crucial. Nevertheless, the architecture should be open in a way to enable easy integration of new processing services. Results of processing services might be directly sent to the client application or be used by following services. Therefore, the architecture should ensure a flexible handling of results. All architecture requirements are listed in Table 7.2.

7.2 Existing NLP Tools and Frameworks

In the field of natural language processing, systems, architectures and frameworks addressing concrete NLP problems have been introduced. OpenCalais [64] is a tool set for NLP and machine learning that allows metatagging of textual information and, in this way, generating semantic content. In addition, a broad range of language processing tool-kits are available (e.g. NLTK [65], MontyLingua [66] or LingPipe [67]). Some of them are working in a pipeline fashion [68, 69]. For example, UAM Text Tools provide command-line programs that realise concrete NLP tasks (e.g. tokenization, sentence splitting, morphologic analysis) which can be connected in various ways [68]. Language processing tools as such are clearly useful, but it is even more relevant to make use of them in more sophisticated systems in general and in healthcare applications in particular. In contrast, showing a way of integrating text analysis methods into healthcare applications in a re-usable manner is our focus in this chapter.

Frameworks for creating modular NLP applications allow arranging modules that perform different tasks of linguistic processing (e.g. tokenization, POS tagging) in a processing pipeline. They target at creating systems for linguists or knowledge engineers, allowing them to create new NLP tools by arranging services in a certain way. Example frameworks are GATE and UIMA.

The Unstructured Information Management Architecture (UIMA [70]) framework is an open, scalable and extendible platform for building text analytics applications or search solutions that process unstructured information. It allows specifying analytic pipelines, describes a set of design patterns and suggests certain data representations. It enables developers to build analytic modules and to compose textanalytic-enabled applications from multiple analytic providers, encouraging collaboration and facilitating value extraction for unstructured information. UIMA was already exploited for analysing and extracting information from clinical text [71].

GATE (General Architecture for Text Engineering, [72]) is both, a framework and graphical environment for human language processing. It enables combining different processing modules and language resources for building a pipeline of NLP components. The framework comprises a Java suite of tools for all sorts of natural language processing tasks, including information extraction in many languages. GATE includes an information extraction system called ANNIE (A Nearly-New Information Extraction System) which is a set of modules comprising a tokenizer, a gazetteer, a sentence splitter, a part of speech tagger, a named entity transducer and a coreference tagger. ANNIE can be used as-is to provide basic information extraction functionality, or provide a starting point for more specific tasks.

Existing frameworks and approaches are focusing either on one concrete textanalytic-enabled application and used service-oriented architectures to realize this application, or they are addressing specific NLP tasks and resist on providing a general architecture for complete application systems. In the following, we present an architecture for a textanalytic-enabled system that provides a more general view on these applications. Single NLP systems or modules as produced with GATE or UIMA can be integrated in the textanalytic-enabled healthcare application as NLP services.

7.3 Architecture for Textanalytic-Enabled Applications

After collecting the requirements, it becomes clear that the principle of a service-oriented architecture could be well suited for designing textanalytic-enabled systems, since single services can be easily integrated and re-used in various applications once the services have been implemented. Service-oriented architecture (SOA) is a software design and software architecture design pattern based on discrete pieces of software providing application functionality as services to other applications. A service is a self-contained unit of functionality. In this way, it is independent of any vendor, product or technology. This enables a flexible way of developing such applications.

In this section, a service-oriented architecture for textanalytic-enabled healthcare applications is described. Figure 7.1 shows the four major components of the architecture. It comprises a *client* facing application and a *server* application acting

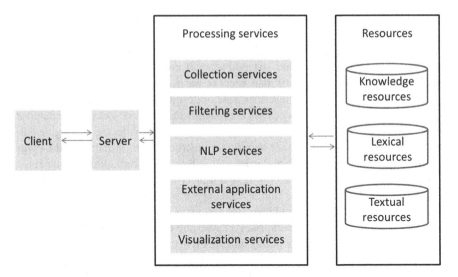

Fig. 7.1 In our service-oriented architecture for textanalytic-enabled applications, four main groups of components can be distinguished: the client, the server, processing services and resources

as a facade to the system. *Processing services* group the computational components, and *resources* encapsulate data that need to be persisted for the system to work properly. Details such as acquiring data from a client application or from multiple data sources of several types are not shown explicitly in the figure and will not be explained in detail. The focus is rather on the components of such architecture. They are described in the following in more depth.

7.3.1   Client

The client might be an existing system such as a web browser, a text processor or any other client. It allows starting functionalities that realise a concrete healthcare scenario. The end-user of the application interacts with the client to make use of the functionalities. Results achieved from the server are made available or accessible through the client.

7.3.2   Server

The server is responsible for the interaction between client and processing services, the invocation of services and the communication with external applications. In its role as service orchestrator it invokes services in the right order and transmits the results of one service as input to the next service if required. It prepares the responses of the processing services, collects the results of the services and transmits the results to the client (e.g. some generated HTML code). Service descriptions that comprise information on input and output of the processing services, required resources, and other prerequisites are maintained by the server. The final visualisation of processing results is realised through the client.

The server also enables communication with other relevant applications. We can distinguish three different kinds of applications with which the server might be interacting in terms of starting applications or collecting data:

- General desktop applications (e.g. open the "send mail" window in E-Mail programs),
- Healthcare applications (e.g. data transfer to the hospital information system, glucose monitoring system), and
- Internet applications (e.g. running a PubMed search).

For some of these applications direct API calls from the server might be sufficient. Other applications may require building custom extensions to allow for interactions with the server (effectively becoming an extended API). To realise communication with external applications, the server receives abstract invocation messages generated by a corresponding processing service (see below, shown as *External Application Services* in Fig. 7.1).

7.3.3 Processing Services

The processing services realise the actual processing. They might be independent from each other or the output from one processing service is required as input for another. We identified five different groups of processing services that are required to realise a textanalytic-enabled application. These include: Data Collection Services, NLP Services, External Application Services, Visualisation Services and Filtering Services. Details are given in the following paragraphs.

Data Collection Services are responsible for collecting (textual) data from different resources, e.g. from web pages, weblog postings (e.g. by a *Web crawling service*) or even data from a user's desktop. Further, results from clinical measurements might be relevant for an application scenario. Thus, data need to be collected from external applications including medical devices (see also External Application Service).

NLP Services provide text analysis functionalities on different levels of granularity. Their main task is to analyse natural language, to identify relevant pieces of information and make them available for follow-up services. NLP services can be grouped into three classes: (1) services for preparing the data for further processing (e.g. string preparation and normalisation or a web page parser to identify text content), (2) services for basic text processing such as general or domain-specific named entity recognition, lexicon look-up, and (3) complex text processing and analysis services. The latter include among others services for sentiment analysis, relationship extraction or document classification, trend analysis or event detection. It is relevant to provide as processing services also modules for more complex NLP tasks since this allows making the system development as easy as possible for system developers even with limited knowledge and experience in developing NLP tools. An example of a complex service is a service that first extracts information on the health status from patient documents and then categorises it as "good/improved", "bad/worsened".

Filtering Services allow filtering identified information and produced results. Filtering criteria may include user specified preferences, a user's working context, his role and responsibility in a healthcare process, access rights to a systems and data etc. One potential filtering service could be a personalisation service that allows restricting presented results to those, a user is interested in or that fit to his current working context. Filtering includes also integration of information from different resources which is relevant to avoid presentation of the same information multiple times.

Application Services are responsible for interaction with external applications. On the one hand, a textanalytic-enabled application should allow for starting another relevant application (e.g. a specific external application such as a text processor with a specific template). On the other hand, it should allow for collecting data stored in external applications like for example in a health information system. Therefore, application services allow creating a formal description of the kind of application that need to be started, collect the required input information and provide details on the expected output. This formal description is then transmitted to the server who takes care of starting an appropriate application and—if required—collects the processing results of that application.

The *Visualisation Services* realise the visualisation and result presentation of the application. Visual alerts, tag clouds, timelines or graph-like representations of data are some options that might be relevant. Additionally, information extracted from different data sources should be integrated in a visual manner for improving readability and perception of the information. An HTML Wrapper is one possible visualisation service that integrates the results of other services into an HTML page. This page can then be shown to the end user through the client.

7.3.4   Resources

Some of the processing services presented before require additional knowledge which is represented in the proposed architecture as resource component. Three different kinds of resources can be distinguished. *Knowledge Resources* contain background knowledge on the domain or a patient (e.g. medication, diagnoses). In the medical domain, there are for example ontologies available where connections between diseases and symptoms are accessible (e.g. SNOMED CT, see Chap. 8). Knowledge resources also include rules for interpreting numerical or any other data (e.g. minimum and maximum values for glucose level) or information on user preferences. *Lexical Resources* provide relevant information mainly for NLP services and comprise for example lists of person names, symptoms, anatomical structures, polarity information etc. Lexical Resources can be used to identify relevant entities through string matching. *Textual Resources* include unstructured background information, for example desktop documents, web documents, clinical documents, clinical guidelines, questionnaires or even links to this kind of resources that are of interest.

7.4 Benefits and Shortcomings

Creating textanalytic-enabled medical applications following the architecture presented in this chapter has several benefits. First, very different applications dealing with various scenarios can be developed by considering this architecture. This is in contrast to the existing tools and frameworks that focused only on single, self-contained systems. Second, the architecture ensures re-use of existing modules. Once a set of processing modules has been implemented, resources only need to be integrated in an appropriate manner to create a textanalytic-enabled healthcare application. Third, the service-oriented structure of the architecture assures flexibility of creating healthcare applications addressing other scenarios by the ability of adding new services. Processing services and resources are strictly separated which allows using the same resources by different processing services. In summary, the architecture offers a computational linguist or system developer a workflow environment that allows her or him to rapidly prototype and test applications built from services and resources specified by the architecture.

With respect to the collected requirements the following observations can be made: due to the client—server structure, textanalytic-enabled medical applications developed using the suggested architecture can be integrated into any client application. Further, the user context is considered by using different filtering services. Analysis and extraction is realised by implementations of corresponding NLP services. External Application Services and Data Collection Services support in realizing data exchange and communication. Therefore, the user requirements are fulfilled by the architecture. This also holds true for the requirements for system developers. The service-oriented architecture enables creating systems with services working in a processing pipeline. Services perform concrete tasks or address solving of concrete problems (e.g. detecting opinions) and are separate from each other which enables easy reuse of components. In this way, for creating a concrete textanalytic-enabled medical application system, implementation details of single services are not required. A system developer does not need to have high competence in knowledge engineering and text analysis methods. This facilitates the implementation process and reduces the required knowledge for creating such applications.

Regarding system requirements, the architecture is open for integration of new services. A flexible handling of results is ensured by allowing further processing of results of single processing services, communication of results to the client application or their use in additional external applications. Since we resisted on discussing implementation details, ensuring the maintenance of resources depends on the final implementation of the architecture. We conclude that the previously collected requirements are fulfilled by the proposed architecture.

The description in this chapter focused on a general architecture and resist on implementation details. We are aware that there are different approaches to realise service-oriented architectures such as WS-* or RESTful. Both may have their benefits and shortcomings when they are used for implementing the proposed architecture.

Chapter 8
Information Extraction from Medical Social Media

Extracting information from unstructured texts is important since automatic processing and analysis of texts requires structured information. Algorithms and tools are already available for mapping clinical and biomedical documents to concepts of medical terminologies and ontologies. Once applied to a document they provide extracted concepts that represent the content of a document. However, the question is whether these tools are applicable to medical social media. As we have seen in the previous sections, language in medical social media texts differs from language in clinical documents. In this chapter, we will assess the extraction quality of such tools through a qualitative study. The mapping quality of two mapping or named entity recognition tools originally designed for processing clinical texts is compared when they are applied to medical social media text.

8.1 Problem Description: Extraction of Medical Concepts

Extracting concepts (such as drugs, symptoms, and diagnoses) from clinical narratives constitutes a basic enabling technology to unlock the knowledge within texts and support more advanced reasoning applications such as diagnosis explanation, disease progression modelling, and intelligent analysis of the effectiveness of treatment [73]. Concept extraction from medical social media data is an upcoming important task. Relevant information needs to be extracted and represented in an adequate manner, allowing future processing. Given the huge amount of social media data available, it is clear that automatic methods are required to extract and analyse the content and enable processing. Methods from the following areas are exploited when searching for relevant information in texts:

© Springer International Publishing Switzerland 2015
K. Denecke, *Health Web Science*, Health Information Science,
DOI 10.1007/978-3-319-20582-3_8

Table 8.1 Input and output of information retrieval, information extraction and text mining systems

Method	Input	Output
Information retrieval	Set of documents, search query	Relevant documents matching the query
Information extraction	Set of documents and categories for which information is searched	Extracted data assigned to the categories
Text mining	Set of documents	Information implicitly contained in the texts

- Information retrieval (IR),
- Information extraction (IE),
- Text mining,
- Query-answering,
- Text summarization.

We want to distinguish information retrieval, from information extraction and text mining. Table 8.1 presents the differences of the three methods by means of their input and output.

Information retrieval methods identify relevant documents from document collections based on keywords or query terms [74]. Text mining methods discover new information that is contained implicitly in texts [75]. This includes for example the discovery of previously unknown implications, i.e. when the processing starts, the nature of the result is still unknown. We will concentrate in the following on information extraction while information retrieval is considered in Chap. 12. Information extraction identifies task-specific information in texts and structures that information. The following definition from Cowie and Lehnert [76] covers exactly in what sense we will use the term information extraction throughout this book.

Definition: Information extraction is the identification, and consequent or concurrent classification and structuring into semantic classes, of specific information found in unstructured data sources, such as natural language text, making the information more suitable for information processing tasks.

An information extraction system is specialised on a specific domain (e.g. medicine) [77]. It requires lexical resources, that provide background knowledge and associated terms as well as domain knowledge. In the medical domain, multiple standardized vocabularies and ontologies are available (see Sect. 8.2.2). This knowledge is exploited by extraction tools to identify meanings in sentences and to identify relevant text snippets given an extraction task. Further, knowledge for interpreting the data is necessary. Figure 8.1 shows input and output of an information extraction system as well as necessary resources.

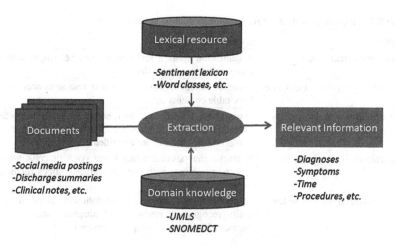

Fig. 8.1 Information extraction process and its underlying resources with examples

8.2 Tools and Resources for Information Extraction

This section provides an overview on information extraction in general and its processing steps. Relevant medical ontologies used as basis for such tools in the domain of medicine are described and the state of the art of information extraction from medical and biomedical documents is summarized.

8.2.1 Information Extraction Process

Information extraction identifies facts or information in texts [78]. An information extraction system is composed of several modules, normally working in a pipeline fashion [72]. Realisation of the single modules depends on the system.

The processing on text-, word- and sentence-level (see Table 8.2) can be seen as linguistic analysis of a text and is required as preprocessing for the actual information extraction process. Domain analysis comprises named entity recognition, coreference resolution, relation extraction and template filling. Named-entity recognition (NER) aims at identifying within a collection of text all of the instances of a name for a specific type of thing [79]. Examples of named entities include names of diseases and illnesses, drugs, persons, or locations. Recognised entities can be mapped to concepts to enable a normalised representation of extracted information.

A concept represents a single meaning. Due to the flexibility in language usage, the same meaning can be expressed in different ways, e.g. through a noun, its synonym, an abbreviation etc. Through mapping of terms to concepts of a terminology, texts can be represented semantically and become interpretable

Table 8.2 Processing modules of information extraction systems

Module	Explanation
Tokenization (text-level)	Tokenization splits a text into tokens, i.e. single words. Dates and numbers are detected
Sentence detection (sentence-level)	Sentence detection structures a text into sentences, item lists, table contents etc.
Lexical and morphological analysis (word-level)	During the lexical and morphological analysis, word classes and lexical features are assigned to terms in sentences. Named entities are identified
Syntactic analysis (phrase-level)	Syntactic analysis determines larger syntactic constituents (e.g. noun phrase, verb phrase) and determines relations between them
Domain analysis (template-level)	Domain analysis consists of the following steps: named entity recognition, resolution of anaphora and coreferences, construction of template elements

for computer algorithms. For example, the UMLS Metathesaurus (see below) is organised by concepts: each concept has specific attributes defining its meaning. It is linked to the corresponding concept names in the various source vocabularies. Entities can be recognised in natural language text in two ways:

1. Simple lexicon lookup; and
2. Extraction patterns that are either manually created or learnt from training corpora using supervised machine learning techniques.

Lexicon lookup approaches search for matches with words of a lexicon of named entities in a given text. Difficulties are found to arise, namely because there is no complete dictionary for most types of medical or biomedical entities. Therefore, the simple text-matching algorithms that are commonly used in other domains are not sufficient here. In extraction pattern-based approaches, patterns such as "[Title] [Person]" for the extraction of a person name (e.g. "Mr. Warren") are generated either by hand or by supervised machine learning techniques. Manual rule-based approaches can be very efficient, but unfortunately such systems require manual efforts to produce the rules that govern them. Machine learning techniques on the other hand that don't require costly human annotators do however require large training corpora to train their underlying models.

Resolution of co-references deals with identifying expressions that refer to the same entity (e.g. pronouns). Relation extraction comprises the extraction of links between entities. In Chap. 9 an approach to relation extraction will be introduced and evaluated. Template filling is another subtask within the information extraction domain analysis and considers the aggregation of extracted concepts, named entities and relations into a given template.

8.2.2 Medical Ontologies

As mentioned previously, information extraction requires formalized domain-knowledge and lexical resources. In the medical domain, many vocabularies exist. We will describe three terminologies in more depth that are frequently exploited within medical information extraction systems.

The **Unified Medical Language System (UMLS [80])** is composed of three main knowledge components: Metathesaurus, Semantic Network and SPECIALIST Lexicon.

- The UMLS Metathesaurus integrates vocabularies from the biomedical domain (e.g., MeSH, SNOMED CT) and provides a mapping structure between them. Each concept has specific attributes that define its meaning. In the release version 2013AB, the Metathesaurus comprises 2,930,638 concepts in 21 languages [80]. The vocabularies that are integrated into the UMLS contribute thesaural relationships between concepts (e.g., "child" or "parent" relationships). Each concept is assigned to at least one semantic type of the Medical Semantic Network (MSN).
- The UMLS MSN [81] is a network of general semantic categories or types where semantic types are linked by relationships. It provides 134 semantic types that have been aggregated into a set of 15 semantic groups to reduce complexity [82] (e.g. the concept atrial fibrillation belongs to the semantic types *Finding and Pathologic Function* that in turn belong to the semantic group *Disorders*). Semantic network relationships connect UMLS semantic types to each other. For example associate the relations labeled *location_of, has_location* and *adjacent_to* the semantic type *Body Part, Organ, or Organ Component* with the semantic type *Body Location or Region*.
- The SPECIALIST Lexicon provides linguistic knowledge. For example, syntactical information on (medical) terms, and natural language processing tools, such as a tokenizer which splits a sentence into tokens are part of the SPECIALIST Lexicon.

As mentioned before, the UMLS integrates various vocabularies including MeSH and SNOMED CT. **MeSH (Medical Subject Headings)** is the controlled vocabulary thesaurus of the National Library of Medicine which is used for indexing articles for their digital library known as PubMed. MeSH consists of sets of terms, naming descriptors in a hierarchical structure. There are 26,853 descriptors in 2013 MeSH. There are also over 213,000 entry terms that assist in finding the most appropriate MeSH Heading, for example, "Vitamin C" is an entry term to "Ascorbic Acid." In addition to these headings, there are more than 214,000 headings called Supplementary Concept Records (formerly Supplementary Chemical Records) within a separate thesaurus [83]. At the most general levels of the hierarchical structure are the very broad headings, such as "Anatomy" or "Mental Disorders". More narrowly defined headings for these general terms are found at the more restricted levels of the hierarchy. For example, terms such as "Ankle" and "Conduct Disorder" reflect refinements of the categories of anatomy and mental disorders, respectively.

SNOMED CT (Systematized Nomenclature of Medicine [84]) is a multilingual collection of medical terms. It contains more than 311,000 active concepts with unique meanings and formal logic-based definitions organized into hierarchies and around one million relationships. SNOMED CT provides general terminology for the electronic health record, consisting of concepts, descriptions and relationships:

- *Concepts* represent clinical ideas, such as "neoplasm" or "abscess",
- *Descriptions* link appropriate human-readable terms to concepts,
- *Relationships* link each concept to other concepts that have a related meaning. As such, relationships provide formal definitions as well as other characteristics of concepts.

SNOMED CT is owned, maintained and distributed by the International Health Terminology Standard Development Organisation (IHTSDO). It is a standard clinical terminology with specific support for multi-lingual translation and is now in use in more than 50 countries.

8.2.3   Information Extraction Tools for Medical and Biomedical Texts

For extracting diagnoses or medical procedures, specialised tools were developed that are described in the following. Stanford NLP tools [85], Alchemy API, LingPipe or OpenCalais are some examples for NLP tools that can be exploited for developing text analysis systems. However, these systems were mainly designed for processing news articles and often specifically trained on news data sets. Within named entity recognition, these tools support detection of entities referring to persons, organization or locations.

Existing information extraction systems designed for processing clinical documents or biomedical literature are based on

- Pattern matching techniques such as regular expressions (e.g. the REgenstrief eXtraction tool [86]),
- Full or partial parsing (e.g. LifeCode system [87]), or
- A combination of syntactic and semantic analysis (e.g. MedLEE [88] and MetaMap [89]).

They were mainly developed to extract information from textual documents in the electronic health record, among others from chest radiography reports, radiology reports, echo-cardiogram reports and discharge summaries. Evaluations showed that the current natural language processing tools for clinical narratives are effectively enough for practical use [90].

In the following, two tools that were developed to process clinical text or biomedical literature are described in more depth. These tools are free available and form the basis for our quantitative study of extraction quality from medical social media texts.

The Apache Clinical Text Analysis and Knowledge Extraction System (**cTAKES**, [91]) is an open-source natural language processing system for extracting information from documents. The algorithms were specifically trained to process clinical documents in the electronic medical record. Among others, it provides a named entity recognizer that identifies clinical named entities in text using a dictionary-lookup algorithm. The recognition concentrates on concepts of specific semantic types: diseases, sign/symptoms, procedures, anatomy and drugs. cTAKES was built using the Apache UIMA Unstructured Information Management Architecture engineering framework (see Sect. 7.2) and the OpenNLP natural language processing toolkit [92]. Its components are specifically trained for the clinical domain out of diverse manually annotated datasets, and create rich linguistic and semantic annotations that can be utilised by clinical decision support systems and clinical research. cTAKES has been used in a variety of use cases in the domain of biomedicine such as phenotype discovery, translational science, pharmacogenomics and pharmacogenetics. In evaluations with clinical notes, the algorithm achieved F-scores from 0.715 to 0.76 for the NER task [93].

The **MetaMap System** [89] is provided by the National Library of Medicine (NLM). The tool maps natural language text to concepts of the UMLS Metathesaurus. MetaMap uses a knowledge-intensive approach based on symbolic, natural-language processing and computational-linguistic techniques. Besides being applied for both, IR and data-mining applications, MetaMap is one of the foundations of NLM's Medical Text Indexer (MTI) which is being used for both semi-automatic and fully automatic indexing of biomedical literature at NLM. MetaMap was originally developed to extract information from MEDLINE abstracts, but has been applied to clinical documents as well (e.g. for pathology reports [94], for respiratory findings [95]).

MetaMap follows a lexical approach and works in several steps. First, it parses a text into paragraphs, sentences, phrases, lexical elements and tokens. From the resulting phrases, a set of lexical variants is generated. Candidate concepts for the phrases are retrieved by lexicon lookup from the UMLS Metathesaurus and evaluated. The best candidates are organised into a final mapping in such a way as to best cover the text. Precision of MetaMap, which is the fraction of retrieved concepts that are relevant, was assessed for different text types already, namely for respiratory findings [95], mailing lists [96] and figure captions in radiology reports [97]. The precision for these text types ranges between 56 and 89.7 %.

8.3   Extracting Medical Concepts from Medical Social Media: A Qualitative Study

For online news, a comparison of several NER tools (e.g., Alchemy API, DBpedia Spotlight, OpenCalais etc.) has already been performed [98]. Similar comparisons of NER tools for medical social media have not yet been made. Further, evaluation results of NER tools in the medical domain are only available for extraction from clinical or biomedical texts and still unavailable for medical social media. On the other hand, reliable technologies for analysing the textual content of medical social media are necessary. In this section, we describe results of a qualitative comparison of two clinical named entity recognition tools, cTAKES, MetaMap, when they are applied to medical social media documents. The objective is to clarify whether the tools extract relevant information from social media correctly and to determine which information remains unconsidered. The results of the study are important for the development of social media processing tools, in particular to decide whether existing technology is sufficient or whether and which adaptations are necessary to achieve good analysis results.

8.3.1   Study Design

We applied the two tools to (1) ten texts drawn from "Health Day News" [99] and (2) ten blog postings from "WebMD" [40] selected from the MSM dataset (see Sect. 3.3). Each text comprises approximately 500 words. The mapping results produced by MetaMap and cTakes when applied to the data set were checked manually, sentence by sentence by two persons, a computer scientist specialised in medical informatics and a medical doctor. The assessment of the output of the tools concerned the correctness of the extraction, the relevance of the extracted concepts and limitations and possibilities of the extraction tools with respect to processing medical social media data. More specifically, the annotators had to judge the

- Presence of the detected named entity (present in the text or not),
- Relevance of the detected named entity (relevant or irrelevant), and
- Type of the detected named entity (correct or incorrect).

We identified words that are crucial for understanding the text or sentence which could not be identified by either one of the tools used. Correct and incorrect annotations were counted. Extracted concepts were labeled as *wrong* when they did not represent the actual meaning of the underlying term or even when the extraction was incomplete (e.g. when for the phrase *breast cancer* only the concept referring to *breast* is provided). Further, observations on reasons for errors were collected.

The objective of the assessment is to give insights into the possibilities and limitations of these tools when they are applied to medical social media data. Unfortunately, the systems use different versions of the UMLS. MetaMap was run

Table 8.3 cTakes categories and MetaMap correspondings

cTakes category	MetaMap categories
Diseases	Disease or syndrome; acquired abnormality
Sign/symptom	Sign or symptom; physiologic function; laboratory or test result; injury or poisoning
Procedures	Therapeutic or preventive procedure; laboratory procedure; diagnostic procedure
Anatomy	Body system; body substance; body space or junction; body part, organ, or organ component; body location or region; anatomical structure
Drugs	Pharmacologic substance; clinical drug

Table 8.4 Accuracy values per category for both systems

Category	MetaMap (%)	cTakes (%)
Disease	59.6	92.9
Sign, symptom	75.2	92.9
Procedure	69.05	93.7
Anatomy	54.08	98.1
Drug	66.54	93.8

with UMLS 2013AB, while cTAKES is distributed with UMLS 2011AB. However, this is not supposed to have to critically influence the mapping quality in our study.

MetaMap processing was restricted to identify concepts of semantic types that are referring to medical conditions, procedures, medications or anatomy. This restriction was made to achieve comparability with the cTakes results. CTakes only determines concepts referring to these semantic types. More specifically, MetaMap processing was restricted to the semantic types listed in Table 8.3 with their corresponding categories in cTakes.

8.3.2 Mapping Observations

This section describes the evaluation results and observations of the annotators. Accuracy values determined in the evaluation are listed in Table 8.4. cTakes achieved an average accuracy of 94 % for the data set. Annotations of type *DiseaseDisorder, SignSymptom, Drug and Procedure* are correct with around 93 %; and *Anatomy* annotations correct with an accuracy of 98 %.

Compared to the cTakes results, MetaMap's results are more often incomplete and wrong. Symptoms are recognized best with an accuracy of 75.1 %, followed by concepts referring to *procedures* with 69 % accuracy. The accuracy values are significantly lower than those of cTakes. One problem of MetaMap is that certain phrases such as *breast cancer* are not mapped to a disease or finding. Only the location (e.g. *breast*) is annotated. The annotators were asked to consider such mappings as incorrect.

Table 8.5 Proportion of extracted concepts per category

Category	MetaMap (%)	cTakes (%)
Disease	17.5	35.7
Sign, symptom	12.6	27.1
Procedure	28.8	19.1
Anatomy	19.2	15.5
Drug	21.9	2.4

Table 8.5 shows the proportion of extracted concepts per category. The tools show clear differences. cTakes extracted in total 1399 concepts. Half of them are referring to diagnoses and signs and symptoms. In contrast, MetaMap extracted 1020 concepts from the same data set and the majority of concepts refer to procedures and medication.

8.4 Error Analysis and Open Issues

8.4.1 Mapping Errors

The results show, that there are linguistic structures and terms that are well processed by the two tools, mainly explicit mentions of clinical concepts and nouns. Terms from common language or consumer health vocabulary referring to medical concepts are often mapped incorrectly by MetaMap or are even missing in the mapping altogether. Wrong mappings occur in particular for personal pronouns: "I" is mapped to "Iodides [Inorganic Chemical]"; "my" is mapped to "Malaysia [Geographic Area]"; and "she" is mapped to "SHE gene [Gene or Genome]". Verbs are often not mapped at all or are wrongly mapped. For example, the verb "found" in the sentence *Keratin is found in your hair* is mapped to (clinical) "Finding"; or the verb "go" is mapped to the concept "GORAB gene [Gene or Genome]". Keeping the meaning of verbs after mapping is extremely important for interpreting a text automatically (and also manually).

Adjectives were also incorrectly mapped by MetaMap or, like verbs, adjectives may not mapped at all as in "nasty" or "embarrassing" which can drop off the mapping altogether. Another class of wrongly mapped lexical items is that of words or word phrases used in free text (non-clinical texts) which are errantly mapped to clinical phrases. Some of the most common errors are words or word phrases such as "of course" which is mapped to "Course [Temporal Concept]", "Hi" which is mapped to "ABCC8 gene [Gene or Genome]", or "Thanks" which is mapped to "TNFSF13B wt Allele [Gene or Genome]". In addition, numeric expressions can confuse mapping programs as they require separate processing. MetaMap, for example, destroys the expression "about two to 2 1/2 months" which is mapped to two concepts: "Two [Quantitative Concept]" and "month [Temporal Concept]").

Other errors occur in both systems. It could be recognised that named entities referring to job positions, journals, or organizations used in the texts led to wrong or rather misleading annotations in both tools. For example from the phrase *director of the virus hepatitis program* the phrase *virus hepatitis* is annotated as disease occurrence. The term *division* in phrase *a member of the faculty at the division of global health at the University of California* is annotated as *Procedure Mention*.

Anatomical concepts occur sometimes in common language expressions, e.g. *don't have to go hand in hand*. The term *hand* in this phrase is annotated with the category *anatomical site mention* which is correct in general, but in that particular phrase no anatomical concept is meant. Another observation is that the annotation normally concentrates on medical concepts and looses the context. For example, cTakes annotates the phrase *drop in estrogen levels* with a concept referring to *estrogen level*, but the information captured in the complete phrase that—this level is dropping—is lost by such annotation since "dropping" is not at all mapped to a concept and thus disappears in the set of concepts that represents a sentence. Another example is the annotation of the phrase *lack of sleep* where the annotation misses *lack*. Given the fact that cTakes concentrates on extraction of medical concepts of selected types, it is not surprising that also qualitative judgements such as *It's a very effective treatment* remain unconsidered in the mapping.

8.4.2   Discussion of Applicability of MetaMap and cTakes on Social Media

Both tools often fail in mapping or produce wrong mappings for verbs, personal pronouns, adjectives and connecting words. Clearly, these terms or at least their meaning and the relationships they infer, are relevant for interpreting the content of a sentence and text. Since persons are describing their own personal experiences and observations in medical social media data, the language they use inevitably includes to a large extent verbs that describe activities of persons and personal pronouns; consequently, it is crucial not to lose the meaning of these personal accounts from patients or healthcare professionals while engaging in automatic processing of blog or forum content. Whereas missing or wrong mappings are not necessarily an algorithmic problem, they might be a problem of the underlying knowledge resource. For example, there is no concept representing the verbs *warn, recommend, cause* or for the adjectives *horrible, miserable, or ineffective* in the UMLS, the language resource on which the tested tools based. This is due to the fact that the terminology has been developed to formalize clinical knowledge, and thus the meanings of verbs or adjectives that are commonly used in medical social media are unfortunately not covered by this terminology.

One must take into consideration that authors of medical social media content often have no medical training. As a result they often do not use the proper medical terms, but paraphrase these concepts instead. People frustrated with their medical conditions may use a metaphor to refer to their maladies. For example, a cancer patient wrote: *The beast is going to kill me.* While the metaphor "beast" is not normally considered as synonym for cancer, this is what the patient used to refer to his illness.

Yet another problem is that MetaMap often provides multiple mappings which may differ significantly in regard to the underlying concepts. The reason for this is that different meanings of words result in various mappings to concepts with different semantic types. No doubt, having multiple mappings available becomes a problem since a system need to select automatically the correct one. MetaMap provides confidence values for these different mappings. Nevertheless, when there are several mappings with the same confidence value, it remains a question of how to select the "correct" mapping automatically.

In summary, both tools are able to extract concepts from medical social media when medical conditions or procedures are explicitly mentioned and described by nouns. Concepts extracted by cTakes are mostly correct. The content of the documents can be well described through the extracted concepts. While medical terms are mostly reflected in MetaMap mappings, descriptive or concept-relating words are missing.

8.4.3 Improvements of NER Tools for Processing Medical Social Media

The results of the analysis presented before showed that extraction tools that rely upon biomedical ontologies can be exploited to mine medical social media postings. Several improvements can likewise be made to mapping tools that are used in the medical social media setting: (1) By including general terminological resources such as WordNet, meanings of adjectives could be recognized and considered in the analysis. (2) Another possibility against wrong mappings of medical social media postings is to enhance the underlying ontology by consumer health vocabulary, but this must be done cautiously as it is a very complicated process and could probably lead to problems in processing professional language. (3) A third possibility for an improved mapping or for improved named entity recognition is the extension of the mapping algorithm. Aronson et al. [100] showed that it is possible to apply successfully an ensemble of classification systems originally developed to process medical literature on clinical reports. Such approaches need to be assessed in the future to develop a better suited mapping tool for medical social media. (4) Methods or terminologies need to be extended to be able to recognize metaphors or paraphrases.

In fact, various mapping tools could be used together to achieve a more complete extraction and annotation. Our evaluation showed that existing tools for NER from medical texts fail in extracting mentions of organization or person names. Recognising person and organisation names in advance could help in reducing errors in concept mapping to clinical concepts. The named entities referring to persons and organisations could be filtered out before processing. Further, open information extraction techniques [101] could help in identifying relevant relations as they are expressed by verbs in medical social media. This extraction paradigm learns a general model of how relations are expressed based on unlexicalized features such as part-of-speech tags (e.g., the identification of a verb in the surrounding context) and domain-independent regular expressions (e.g., the presence of capitalization and punctuation). By making use of such extraction techniques, it would no longer be necessary to specify in advance the relevant terms or patterns found in social media. This approach may prove more practical given the fact that medical postings are fast-changing, thus making it simply impossible to continuously update the language of social media and their underlying lexical resources manually. Such an approach of open information extraction could help to identify relations expressed by verbs in medical social media without specifying in advance relation types of interest. To avoid wrong mappings of personal pronouns or connecting words, negative lists could be exploited, i.e. lists that instruct the algorithms not to map the listed words at all.

8.4.4 Discussion of the Study Design

Some limitations of this study have to be mentioned. Since a reference standard is missing for the task under consideration, the evaluation was done manually and only on a few texts derived from two different blogs. It might be that other blog authors are writing in a completely different style, using for example medical terminology in a similar way than it is done in clinical narratives. Further, we did not determined an interannotator agreement since the annotators assessed different texts. Recall of the mapping would be also interesting to analyse. MetaMap provides mapping candidates and sometimes provides multiple, ranked mappings. We considered in the evaluation the best mapping or the first one in the list when multiple mappings had the same rank. It might be, that the correct mapping was not the first one and was thus not considered in the assessment.

We did not compare the mappings of the two tools directly, i.e. it was not identified to what extent the tools provided the annotation to the same words. Such comparison would be interesting for future analysis. cTakes provides additional annotations, such as verbs. They were not considered in the presented analysis.

Chapter 9
Relation Extraction

Relationships semantically connect entities and thus it is crucial to identify them when analysing texts in order to understand and interpret the content correctly. Only with extracted relations, a deeper text understanding (e.g., recognising the who, when, where of a medical event and the temporal and causal relationships between events) is possible. We have seen in the analysis of the medical social media language in Chap. 6 and in the analysis of mapping quality of existing information extraction tools, that more complex sentence structures occur in medical social media data. The tools failed in analysing meanings of verbs, which would be crucial to automatically analyse and process this data for example for knowledge gathering or generating semantic structures from medical social media. In this chapter, we will describe one possible approach to relation extraction coming from the field of Web Mining and study its relevance and performance on medical social media texts.

9.1 Extracting Relationships: Definitions and Approaches

A (semantic) relation is defined as a predicate ranging over two arguments, where an **argument** represents concepts, objects or people in the real world and the **relation predicate** describes the association or interaction that holds between the concepts represented by the arguments. Consider for example the sentence *Frozen section exam showed a fibroadenoma with some proliferative hyperplasia within the fibroadenoma*. It contains several relations, e.g. the relation *showed* (*Frozen section exam - showed - a fibroadenoma*). Another relation that could be labelled *accompanied by* exist between *fibroadenoma* and *some proliferative hyperplasia*. Relationships semantically connect the entities and thus it is crucial to identify them when analysing texts in order to understand the content.

© Springer International Publishing Switzerland 2015
K. Denecke, *Health Web Science*, Health Information Science,
DOI 10.1007/978-3-319-20582-3_9

Table 9.1 Example relation types from surgical reports

Observation	Activity
Appeared, showed, revealed, has, presented	Vacuumed with, abraded, carried down, closed, cooled, brought, approximated, divided, elevated, entered, extracted, made, harvested, injected, instilled, placed, rotated, removed, irrigated

We can distinguish semantic and temporal relations. A temporal relation describes the ordering in time of events or states. In this work, we focus on determining semantic relations. On the other hand, relations can be characterised based on their relation type (e.g., relation of type *has_finding* or *has_location*). For example, we can distinguish relations describing observations and relations describing activities. Observations can concern the patient (e.g. *The patient tolerated the procedure well* or *The patient desires a vasectomy.*) or medical conditions (e.g. *External hemorrhoids were found*). Activities comprise surgical activities and administrative or management activities (e.g. *She was scheduled for surgery.*). Some example relation types falling into the two categories *observation* and *activity* are listed in Table 9.1.

Methods for extracting or identifying semantic relationships among terms and concepts were so far only rarely introduced and studied in the medical domain, and in particular for medical social media. Existing approaches to relation extraction require a specification of extraction patterns. This means that it needs to be known in advance which relation can exist between entities in a text and how it is characterised. Relations such as a *treat*-relation (as in *Insulin treats diabetes*) can be specified in advance. However, there are other relations in medical texts that cannot be characterised in advance. For example in surgical reports relations are expressed that are normally difficult to characterise in advance since they describe the real procedure as it happened. Even though procedures will be repeated for the same surgical interventions, there might be complications or interactions that are unique. Further, semantic relations can be described in different words.

In the field of Web Mining, **open information extraction** was introduced as possible solution to process web documents. Open information extraction (open IE, [61, 102]) is the task of extracting assertions from massive corpora without requiring a pre-specified vocabulary. It identifies phrases that denote relations in sentences. The extraction avoids the problem of being restricted to a pre-specified vocabulary. Existing approaches (TextRunner [101], WOEpos WOEparse [103], ReVerb [61]) concentrate on extracting binary relations of the form (argument 1, relation phrase, argument 2). They label sentences automatically with extractions using heuristics; a relation phrase extractor is learnt using a sequences-labelling graphical model and from each sentence, candidate pairs of nominal phrase (NP) arguments are identified. Then, the learnt extractor is applied to label each word between the two phrases as part of the relation phrase or not. TextRunner [101], for example, uses a Naive Bayes model with unlexicalized parts of speech and NP-chunk features, trained using examples from the Penn Treebank. Other systems use syntactic patterns based on verbs to extract relation phrases that are determined through a full dependency parse [104]. Even though, open IE is domain-independent, these particular methods were so far only rarely considered in the medical domain. In the following, we will apply ReVerb, one of the open IE systems, to a set of surgical reports that are provided wiki-like in the web to study its processing quality and results.

9.2 ReVerb for Medical Relation Extraction

We chose the open information extraction tool ReVerb [61] for our experiments since an improved quality over other open information extraction systems such as TextRunner was reported. ReVerb is designed for web-scale information extraction, where the target relations cannot be specified in advance and speed is important [61].

ReVerb takes as input a sentence tagged with part of speech information and chunks of nominal phrases and returns relation triples consisting of [argument 1, relation phrase, argument 2]. The algorithm works as follows:

1. Relation extraction: For each verb, the longest word sequence is identified that (1) starts with the verb, (2) satisfies the syntactic and lexical constraints.
2. Argument extraction: For each relation phrase identified in step 1, the nearest noun phrase to the left of the relation word (verb) is identified.

The syntactic constraint requires the relation phrase to match a POS pattern. The pattern limits relation phrases to be either (a) a verb, (b) a verb followed immediately by a preposition or (c) a verb followed by nouns, adjectives or adverbs ending in a preposition. ReVerb assigns a confidence score to each extracted relation depending on some specified features. Our preliminary assessments showed that this score cannot be used reliably to select correctly extracted relations. Therefore, we ignored the confidence score in our experiments.

Our objective of relation extraction is not only to extract relation triples in the sense of linking phrases, but to generate a standard representation reflecting the links between medical concepts. For this purpose, we exploit ReVerb in a processing pipeline:

1. A text is structured into sentences using the OpenNLP Sentence Splitter trained with an English sentence model.
2. Each detected sentence is processed by ReVerb (instead of the complete text). Further, paragraph introducing words are removed before entering the relationship extraction process (e.g. the heading *Preoperative Diagnosis* is removed from the sentence)
3. ReVerb is applied to extract relation triples.
4. Extracted relations are normalized: The relation arguments are mapped to UMLS concepts using MetaMap[89]. The relation type is normalized by stemming.

The result of this pipeline is still a triple, but the arguments consist of UMLS concepts and the relation type is a stemmed verb.

9.3   Quality of Relation Extraction

9.3.1   Evaluation Setup and Objectives

In a small study, we analysed the quality of this approach. The evaluation studies the quality of the adapted open information approach on surgical reports derived form the web. The experiments mainly try to answer the following questions:

- Which quality achieves open information extraction on surgical reports?
- What are the possibilities and limitations of the extraction approach?
- Which improvements are necessary?

To address these questions, we perform experiments by applying the methods described before to the surgical report data set (see Sect. 3.3 for details) comprising 471 sentences. The sentence splitting and filtering resulted in 312 sentences for those 24 reports. For each sentence, the extracted relation (if any) was checked manually by the author of this book with respect to correctness of the arguments and extracted relation type. In more detail, for each sentence, it was checked:

- whether a relation with two arguments was described in the sentence,
- whether the relation was detected correctly (i.e. the arguments and relation type are correct),
- whether the extracted arguments were complete (i.e. no meaningful part got lost through argument mapping and extraction).

Reasons for wrong extractions were collected. A relation was considered to be false when one argument phrase or the relation type was incorrectly extracted. For example, from the sentence *The inferior turbinates had some polypoid changes on them* the arguments *The inferior turbinates* and *them* were extracted. The expectation for the extraction was *[The inferior turbinates] - [had] - [some polypoid changes on them]*. The second argument (and correspondingly the relation type) was wrongly identified. The extracted relation is therefore considered wrong.

A relation was considered correct when type and arguments were extracted correctly, but not necessarily complete. Consider the following example: *Ted hose stockings and pneumatic compression stockings were placed on the patient and a Foley catheter was also inserted.* From this sentence, the algorithm extracts as relation: *[pneumatic compression stockings] - [were placed on] - [the patient]*. This extraction is considered correct since the extracted arguments and relation type are correct. In addition to the quality assessment, we analyse and categorize the types of relations and develop a relationship model for the data set.

9.3.2   Relation Types in the Data Set

In the surgical reports that were used in this experiment, we identified mainly four types of relations:

1. Relations describing surgical procedures that were performed at some location, i.e. relation of the form [*Procedure - relation - Location*], e.g. [*Dissection - was carried out around - a firm mass*],
2. Relations describing characteristics or problems with the procedure, i.e. relation of the form [*Procedure - relation - Characteristic/Problem*], [*the cystic duct - was done with - some difficulty*],
3. Relations describing clinical observations, i.e. relation of the form [*Body area or Procedure - relation - Medical Condition*], e.g. [*electrocautery - showed - a fibroadenoma*], or [*The gallbladder - contained - numerous stones*],
4. Relations describing interactions with or reactions of the patient, i.e. relation of the form [*Person - relation - interaction or reaction*], e.g. [*The patient - tolerated - the procedure well*].

Considering all semantic relations described in the surgical reports, we came up with a relation model for surgical texts (see Fig. 9.1). There are mainly five categories of entities that are within the focus of surgical reports: devices, surgical procedures, patient, medical locations, medical conditions. Single sentences in surgical reports describe relations among those groups of entities. Surgical procedures are normally performed with some device and are done in some medical location, e.g. an anatomical structure. Devices can be inserted into medical locations. These relations refer to activities. Beyond, there are observations: Medical conditions are found at some medical location or during some surgical procedure a medical condition was identified. Surgical procedures can have some characteristics (e.g., a procedure was easy to perform or was impossible).

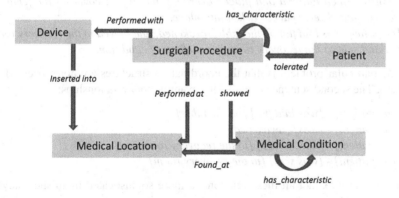

Fig. 9.1 Relation model for surgical reports

Table 9.2 Examples for correct extractions

Sentence	Relation: [Argument 1] - Relation Type - [Argument 2]
The C-arm was rotated to the left	[The C-arm] - was rotated to - [the left]
His O2 saturation remained greater than 90 %	[His O2 saturation] - remained greater than - [90 %]
The posterior capsule remained intact and vacuumed with minimal suction	[The posterior capsule] - vacuumed with - [minimal suction]
The skin was closed in a subcuticular fashion	[The skin] - was closed in [a subcuticular fashion]

9.3.3   Evaluation Results for Relation Extraction

The relation detection identified relations for 252 sentences. 86.1 % of the detected relations were correct. In the sentences where no relation was extracted, a verb or preposition was missing. Thus, the relation was not extracted. This resulted in a recall of 80.1 %. Table 9.2 shows examples for correct extractions.

Errors in relation extraction occurred for the following reasons: (1) complexity of sentences, (2) ambiguity of word classes, and (3) sentence boundary detection. Complex sentence structures are a main reason for wrong (or incomplete) extractions. Typical examples are the following sentences whose syntactical structure is too complex for the extraction approach:

- *Mesh was then tailored and placed overlying the defect, covering the femoral, indirect, and direct spaces, tacked into place.*
- *The patient was laid flat on the table, awakened, and moved to the recovery room bed and sent to the recovery room in satisfactory condition.*

One particular problem is that the coordination structures are not processed by ReVerb. The second sentence contains for example four relationships:

- *[The patient] - [was laid flat] [on the table]*
- *[The patient] - [was] [awakened]*
- *[The patient] - [was moved] [to the recovery room bed]*
- *[The patient] - [was sent] [to the recovery room]*

To correctly extract all these relations, a more sophisticated linguistic analysis is necessary. A second reason for errors are ambiguous words. For example the term *left* is extracted as verb even though it is used as adjective (e.g. as in *left anterior artery*). To address this problem, semantic information could help to resolve ambiguities in determining word classes. Complex sentences and problems in relation extraction also occur when arguments have prepositional attachments. Again dependency trees could help in considering syntactical dependencies in argument extraction.

A last problem to be mentioned as source for errors are enumerations which are problematic for the sentence detector. The sentences are not determined correctly which leads to an input sentence comprising several enumerated items (e.g. *1. Broad-based endocervical poly 2. Broad-based pigmented, raised nevus, right thigh.*).

The quality of extraction with 86.1 % is comparable or even better than results reported elsewhere for relation extraction from clinical texts. However, a comparison to other approaches is difficult since the extraction task is different, and also the textual material underlying the experiments was so far not considered by others.

The recall of the extraction is with 80 % relatively low. A reason for this might be the extraction method of ReVerb. It requires a verb in the sentence—when the verb is missing or no verb is determined, the algorithm does not extract anything. Further, the syntactic constraint requires that the second argument starts or ends with preposition.

Our experiment has some limitations. The annotations were done by only one person. Annotation processes are always subjective. To achieve more objective results, several annotators need to be involved. However, we believe that the results let us recognise the applicability of open information extraction on medical texts. The problem is that no annotated social media data set for this particular problem exists. The extracted relation information can be exploited to train a relation type classifier to distinguish observation relations from activity relations.

Chapter 10
Sentiment Analysis from Medical Texts

Social media data is a huge source of experiences on drugs, treatments, diagnosis etc. This experiential knowledge can provide an extension to the facts and general practices in healthcare treatment. This chapter provides an overview on different facets of sentiment in medical documents in general and in medical social media in particular [63].

Mining sentiments and opinions in medical social media can have multiple applications. Opinions and experiences towards some treatment or drug can be studied for clinical evidence; relations between symptoms, life style and effectiveness can be studied. Positive and negative effects of a treatment can be assessed. Information on the health status and psychological status of a patient can be collected for example by analysing information generated within a patient-doctor social network. Extending sentiment analysis to clinical documents brings additional use cases. Effects of a medication in the treatment of a disease [105] or effects of complications to the outcome of a surgery may be studied. Outcome polarity may be exploited for medical question-answering [106]. But, what exactly is sentiment in medical texts? Which approaches for its automatic analysis do already exist and what are future challenges? Some hints answering these questions will be given in the next sections.

10.1 The Notions of Sentiment in Medicine

Textual information can be broadly categorized into facts and opinions [107]. Facts are objective expressions about entities or events while opinions are usually subjective expressions. They describe people's attitudes, sentiments or feelings towards entities. However, the concept of sentiment or opinion is quite broad. It includes also subjectivity, polarity, emotion or even comparison. While it is

© Springer International Publishing Switzerland 2015
K. Denecke, *Health Web Science*, Health Information Science,
DOI 10.1007/978-3-319-20582-3_10

Table 10.1 Entities and events in the medical domain and possible sentiment characteristics

Entity	Possible sentiment values
Health status	Improve, worsen
Medical condition	Present, improve, worsen
Diagnosis	Certain, uncertain, preliminary
Effect of a medical event	Critical, non-critical
Medical procedure	Positive or negative outcome, successful or unsuccessful
Medication	Helpful, useless, serious adverse events

straightforward that a person can like or dislike a movie or product, sentiment in the context of medicine is difficult to capture with a few words. Facets of sentiment in health-related text can concern (see Table 10.1):

• A **change** in the health status (e.g., a patient can suddenly feel better or worse),
• **Critical events, unexpected situations or specific medical conditions** that impact the patient's life (e.g., *tumour is malignant* as such is a fact, but this medical condition is negative for the patient since it might lead to health problems or death),
• The **outcome or effectiveness of a treatment** (e.g., a surgery can be successfully completed),
• **Experiences or opinions towards a treatment or a sort of drug** (e.g., a patient or a physician can describe serious adverse events after drug consumption),
• The **certainty of a diagnosis** (e.g., a physician can be certain of some diagnosis).

The examples show that *good* and *bad* or *positive* and *negative* in the context of medicine concern the health status, a medical condition or a treatment. It is manifested in improvements or worsenings of certain medical or physical conditions or in the success or failure of a treatment (see Fig. 10.1). In the following, these facets are described in more detail.

Sentiment can be seen as a **reflection of the health status** of a patient which can be *good*, *bad* or *normal* at some point in time. Thus, the health status impacts the quality of life of a patient (e.g., a *severe pain* influences the life of a patient much more than a *slight pain*). By analysing that health status over time, improvements or worsenings in the status can be recognized. In clinical narratives, the health status is expressed either implicitly or explicitly. Implicit descriptions of the health status concern the mentioning of symptoms (e.g. *severe pain, extreme weight loss, high blood pressure*). They require additional content information for a correct interpretation. An explicit description of the health status is reflected through phrases such as *the patient recovered well* or *normal*.

A medical condition can exist, improve or worsen. Thus, sentiment can also be considered as **presence or change of a medical condition**. Sentiment in this context can be implicitly considered as severity of a disease, which again, impacts on life circumstances. A medical condition can have different weights: A chief complaint might impact much more the health status, than another symptom. Further, the

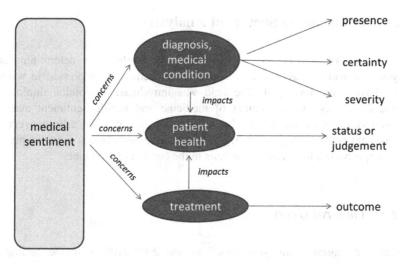

Fig. 10.1 Facets of sentiment in medical contexts: sentiment can concern the patient health, a medical condition or the treatment. For each aspect, sentiment can occur in different shapes

certainty of a diagnosis can be seen as opinion of a physician. For example, a diagnosis can be a suspicion or it can be assured. This opinion on the certainty of a diagnosis impacts the treatment decision: When a diagnosis is certain, a treatment decision can be made; otherwise additional examinations are necessary. Another interesting facet of sentiment concerns the **judgement of medical conditions**, in particular with respect to the severity of a medical condition. For instance, events such as a *bleeding* can be positive or negative, critical or less critical. The phrase *blood pressure decreased* could express a positive or negative change depending on the previous state of blood pressure. A decrease of blood pressure can be good when it was too high before. This also shows that sentiment in clinical narratives cannot always be manifested in single terms of phrases, but the context is important.

Additional sentiment aspects concern the treatment. It can be complex or less complex, urgent or less urgent. The **outcome of a treatment** can be *positive*, *negative* (e.g. surgery was successful or failed), *neutral* or a treatment can have *no outcome*. The outcome can often only be derived from the described effects of a treatment to a medical condition. For example, a statement that a medical condition improved allows to draw the conclusion that the treatment had a positive outcome. **Observations and opinions** towards treatments or medications expressed in clinical narratives or in social media documents provide another facet of sentiment in the context of medicine.

In conclusion, the concept of medical sentiment is very complex and has multiple facets which makes it very interesting, but also challenging for being analysed automatically. In the following, we are reviewing existing approaches to sentiment analysis, collect application areas and technical challenges for medical sentiment analysis.

10.2   Approaches to Sentiment Analysis

In the context of Web Science and Web Mining, methods for determining and analysing subjectivity as well as of opinions and emotions expressed in written format have been developed. The field was introduced as opinion mining, or sentiment analysis. In the context of medicine and health, sentiment analysis increasingly gains in interest. In this section, we first provide a brief overview on sentiment analysis in general. Then, we describe and classify more deeply the existing approaches to sentiment analysis in the context of medicine.

10.2.1   General Overview

Research in sentiment analysis started around 2004 [108] with the mining of opinions in customer reviews and online news. The initial task considered was to distinguish *positive* from *negative* reviews (referred to as **polarity analysis**), or *subjective* from *objective* parts of a text (referred to as **subjectivity analysis**). Later on, additional tasks have been introduced: **emotion analysis** determines the emotional category of texts (e.g. *anger, disgust*) [109, 110] while **intensity analysis** focusses on identifying different levels of polarity or emotion (e.g. *very positive, very sad*).

Existing sentiment analysis methods that have been developed for processing unstructured text in web media, treat the task as classification problem: a classifier is trained to detect the polarity at sentence or document level. For example, Pang et al. have presented a series of supervised methods such as Naïve Bayes, support vector machines and maximum entropy classification [111, 112]. An unsupervised mechanism has been developed by Turney, who proposed a solution to recognize the semantic orientation of texts [113].

These approaches base upon feature sets including semantic or lexical features. Often, the underlying assumption is that sentiment is explicitly mentioned in the text, and is thus manifested in opinionated words. Normally, adjectives, adverbs and specific nouns express sentiments in free texts. Considering this, the conventional sentiment analysis is based on the detection and analysis of such opinionated terms (semantic features). Generally, those terms are categorized into the categories *positive, negative* and *neutral* and made available in sentiment lexicons (see Sect. 10.2.2). The latter are then exploited by sentiment analysis algorithms to identify the opinionated terms and their polarity in a text through lexicon-lookup.

Beyond a lexicon-lookup for identifying opinionated terms, additional features can be extracted from texts for their exploitation in sentiment analysis methods. They include lexical features such as unigrams, bigrams and part of speech.

Sentiment analysis can be considered at different levels: at the level of a word, aspect, sentence and document. Pang et al. [111] considered the problem on document level. However, there is a need for fine-grained approaches to sentiment analysis. Aspect-based analysis aims to identify the aspects of entities and assigns a sentiment to each aspect (e.g. *The CD is good but it was too expensive* describes two aspects, content of the CD and price) [114].

Studies showed that sentiment analysis is often domain-dependent [115] since the polarity of single terms can differ depending on the context they are used in. For that reason, feature models on which machine learning classifier base on, need to be trained on domain-specific data sets. Lexicons need to be adapted to the domain-specific interpretations of words. An approach to domain-independent sentiment analysis was presented by Montejo-Raez et al. [116]. They represented each term in a tweet as a vector of weighted WordNet synsets that are semantically close to the term. The weights were used on SentiWordNet [117] to estimate the polarity.

Limited work is available on sentiment analysis from rather objective texts. Balahur et al. applied sentiment analysis methods to news articles to separate the good and bad news content from the good and bad sentiment expressed on a target and to mark explicit opinions [118]. For this particular text type of news articles, opinion is "conveyed through facts that are interpretable by the emotion they convey" [118]. This is to a certain extent comparable to sentiment analysis in healthcare domain: sentiment can be conveyed through diseases, treatments or medical conditions and their impact on a patient's life quality and health status.

10.2.2   Sentiment Lexicons

Many approaches to sentiment analysis base upon sentiment lexicons. They provide an important basis for recognizing sentiment terms and patterns of sentiment expressions in natural language texts. Existing lexicons are SentiWordNet (SWN) [117], WordNetAffect, General Inquirer[119] and the Subjectivity Lexicon (SL) [60]. They contain words and assigned sentiment scores or classes to single terms. The lexicons can be generated manually or through corpus analysis. They are often not considering the peculiarities and differing meanings of terms when used in different domains or do not explicitly make this information on other domains available. SentiWordNet is one of the most widely used sentiment lexicons. It assigns to each synset of WordNet three sentiment scores: positivity, negativity, objectivity. SentiWordNet contains different meanings of terms. However, it is not specified in which domain a term has another meaning (e.g. when the term *right* is just a location mentioning or used in the sense of "correct"). WordNetAffect [120] provides to a number of WordNet synsets one or more affective labels representing emotional states. Mohammad and Turney [121] developed EmoLex, an emotion lexicon generated by manual annotation through Amazon's Mechanical Turk service. The Subjectivity Lexicon of Wilson et al. [60] contains 8221 single-term subjective expressions associated with their polarity.

Beyond using such general sentiment resources, domain-specific lexica are going to be developed considering the domain-dependency of meanings of words. A high quality multi-dimensional lexicon should include the most representative terms in the domain with their semantic relations and high-level event scheme. The extension of an existing lexicon is the most direct way to cover the domain-specific context. One approach is to increase the lexicon coverage by merging a general lexicon and a domain-specific lexicon.

While the conventional methods have mainly focused on determining explicit sentiment expression, the annotation scheme proposed by Deng et al. [122] considered the benefactive and malefactive events towards the opinionated entities and created an extension of the well-known subjectivity lexicon (MPQA) [60]. More specifically, four types of the goodFor and badFor events (gfbf) have been defined: namely, *destruction, creation, gain or loss, benefit or injury.* The events are represented as a triple of text spans ⟨*agent, gfbf, object*⟩, which indicates some subject (noun) such as a person or an organization has brought some good or bad influence to the object (noun). The implicit opinions expressed by the writer are presented in the scheme.

Goeuriot et al. [123] have merged terms from the general lexicons SentiWordNet and Subjectivity Lexicon [60] together. Afterwards, opinionated terms from drug reviews were extracted to extend the merged lexicons. During the extension, the difference of polarity in the general domain and in the medical domain was analysed. They found out that some words considered generally as *neutral* are opinionated in medical texts. Finally, an evaluation with a simple voting algorithm showed that better results can be achieved using the merged lexicon compared to results achieved with well-known general sentiment lexicons.

Ohana et al. [124] evaluated the performance of sentiment detection using four lexicons: General Inquirer [125], Subjectivity Lexicon [60], SentiWordNet and Moby [126]. The lexicons were applied to texts from six general domain data sets including book reviews, hotel feedback and discussions about music and films. The results showed that the accuracy of the single lexicons depends on the domain. More specifically, SentiWordNet has reached the highest accuracy (65–71 %) in four out of six domains, while the Subjectivity Lexicon has provided the best performance (63–65 %) in the two other domains. One reason for this is the large vocabulary coverage of SentiWordNet.

10.2.3   Sentiment Analysis in Medical Context

Similar to general sentiment analysis approaches, existing research on sentiment analysis in the context of medicine can be grouped according to textual source (e.g. medical web content, biomedical literature, clinical note), task (e.g. polarity analysis, outcome classification), method (e.g. rule-based, machine-learning based) and level (e.g. word level, sentence level). The main approaches are described in more detail in the following.

Sentiment Analysis from the Medical Web

In existing research, sentiment is often considered as polarity, i.e. positive, negative or neutral polarity towards some subject. Such categorization is relevant, when in texts opinions towards some person (e.g. a physician), a medication or a medical device is expressed. However, sentiment can be even more. In contrast to products or persons where sentiment mainly comprises like or dislike towards a person or product, opinions or sentiments towards medications, treatments or even diagnoses sentiments have even more facets and are expressed in different words:

- Opinions on physicians, medical devices, medications,
- Personal feelings on own or someone else health status,
- Complications that occurred,
- Facts vs. experiences with some treatment, diagnosis or drug.

A treatment could be painful, but helped. Complications might have arose, but still the treatment was successful. A diagnosis might be frightening, but not really serious or life-threatening. A drug might have serious side effects. How can we characterise sentiment in medical texts?

It becomes clear that sentiment or opinion in medical social media can be expressed differently than sentiments in news or product reviews. A sentiment can also be described by a symptom reflecting a person's health situation, it is not just a feeling, it is characterised by symptoms, by pathological terms. Since in social media, a mixture of facts and experiences is expressed, it might be necessary to distinguish factual information from experiences.

Most research on sentiment analysis in the domain of medicine is considering web data such as medical blogs or forums for the purpose of mining or studying patient opinions or measuring quality. For example, a method was introduced that separates factual texts from experiential texts [49] to measure content quality and credibility in patient-generated content. Assuming that factual content is better than affective content since more information is given (in contrast to moods and feelings) a system has been developed using subjectivity words and a medical ontology to evaluate the factual content of medical social media.

As in general sentiment analysis, existing approaches to sentiment analysis from medical web data are either machine-learning based [127, 128] or rule-based [129]. Most of the work focused on polarity classification: Xia et al. introduced a multi-step approach to patient opinion classification [128]. Their approach determines the topic and the polarity expressed towards that topic. An F-measure of around 0.67 was reported. Sokolova et al. tested several classifier including Naive Bayes, decision trees and support vector machines (SVM) for sentiment classification of tweets [130]. Texts were represented as bag of words. Two classification tasks were considered: three-classes (positive, negative and neutral) and two classes (positive, negative). The best F-measure of 0.69 was achieved through an SVM classifier.

The focus of the work of Biyani et al. [131] was on determining the polarity of sentiments expressed by users in online health communities. More specifically, they performed sentiment classification of user posts in an online cancer support community (cancer survivors network) by exploiting domain-dependent and domain-independent sentiment features as the two complementary views of a post and use them for post classification in a semi-supervised setting using a co-training algorithm. That work was extended later on with features derived from a dynamic sentiment lexicon, whereas the previous work used a general sentiment lexicon to extract features [132].

Smith et al. [133] studied another perspective of sentiment in patient feedback, which are discourse functions such as *expressive* and *persuasive*. A classifier has been evaluated based on a patient feedback corpus from NHS Choices [46]. The results illustrate that the multinomial Naïve Bayes classifier with frequency-based features can achieve the best accuracy (83.53 %). Further, the results showed that a classification model trained solely on an *expressive* corpus can be applied to the *persuasive* corpus directly and achieve a comparable performance as the training based on the corpus with the same discourse function.

Another interesting application of sentiment analysis was presented by Sharif et al. [134]. Their framework extracts important semantic, sentiment, and affect cues for detecting adverse drug events reported by patients in medical blogs. The approach is able to reflect the experiences of people when they discuss adverse drug reactions as well as the severity and the emotional impact of their experiences.

Na et al. [129] presented a rule-based linguistic approach for sentiment classification of drug reviews. They exploited existing resources for sentiment analysis, namely SentiWordNet and the Subjectivity Lexicon [60] and come up with linguistic rules for classification. Their approach achieved an F-measure of 0.79.

Additional work focused on detecting and analysing emotion in medical web documents. Sokolova and Bobicev [135] considered the categories *encouragement* (e.g. hope, happiness), *gratitude* (e.g. thankfulness), *confusion* (e.g. worry, concern, doubt), *facts*, and *facts+encouragement*. They used the affective lexicon Word-NetAffect [120] for emotion analysis of forum entries and achieved with a Naive Bayes classifier an F-measure of 0.518. Melzi et al. [136] applied an SVM classifier on a feature set comprising unigrams, bigrams and specific attributes to classify sentences into one out of six emotion categories.

Sentiment Analysis from Biomedical Literature

In addition to medical social media data, biomedical literature has been analysed with respect to the outcome of a medical treatment. In this context, sentiment refers to the outcome of a treatment or intervention. Four classes were considered in existing work: *positive, negative, neutral outcome* and *no outcome* [137]. Niu et al. exploited a supervised method to classify the (outcome) polarity at sentence level. Uni-grams, bi-grams, change phrases, negations and semantic categories were employed as features. According to the results, the usage of category information and context information derived from a medical terminology, the unified medical language system (UMLS), improved the accuracy of the algorithm.

Sarker et al. developed a new feature called the relative average negation count (RANC) to calculate polarity with respect to the number and position of the negation [138]. This count suggests that a larger total number of negations reflects a negative outcome. The experimental corpus was collected from medical research papers, which are related to the practice of evidence-based medicine. An N-gram feature set with RANC exploited by an SVM classifier achieved an accuracy of 74.9 %.

Sentiment Analysis from Other Medical Texts

Some researchers concentrated on additional sources of medical text for applying sentiment analysis or emotion detection methods. A comprehensive shared task of sentiment analysis based on suicide notes was addressed in an i2b2 challenge [139]. The best performance of an F_1 measure of 0.61 was achieved with an SVM classifier and pattern matching. However, only part of the participating teams of the challenge have published the details of their feature engineering and selection of algorithms.

Cambria et al. [140] introduced Sentic PROMs, a concept where emotion analysis methods were integrated in a framework for measuring healthcare quality. In a questionnaire, patients answered questions regarding their health status. From the entered free text, emotion terms such as "happy" and "sad" were detected using the semantic resources ConceptNet [141] and WordNet-Affect (WNA) [120]. The extractions were assigned to one out of 24 affective clusters following the concept of *hourglass of emotions* [142]. This concept presents the affective common sense knowledge in terms of a vector, which shows the location in the affective space.

10.2.4 Summary of Medical Opinion Mining Approaches

In summary, existing methods for sentiment analysis in the medical domain focused on processing web content or biomedical literature. The clinical narratives which are used to record the activities and observations of physicians as well as patient records have not yet been analysed in that context. In terms of methods, rule-based approaches were presented, but the majority of papers reports on machine-learning methods (SVM [139], Naïve Bayes [130], regression tree) using features such as part of speech, uni-, bi- and tri-grams. General sentiment lexicons are exploited, but experiments showed that they are not well suited for capturing the meanings in medical texts. In contrast to "normal" sentiment analysis, additional domain-specific features have been explored in some approaches, mainly UMLS concepts reflecting medical conditions and treatments. The main tasks considered have been polarity classification, but new tasks are coming up including outcome classification, information content classification or emotion analysis. However, the existing work on medical sentiment analysis is not at all covering all facets of sentiment analysis that we described in Sect. 10.1. In summary, there is still a huge potential for future research. We will outline the main challenges in Sect. 10.4. Table 10.2 summarizes the related work in medical sentiment analysis.

10.3 Application Areas

Sentiment analysis can be applied in the medical domain in multiple ways. We have seen in the related work, that most of the work concentrated on processing medical web documents. Reported applications are:

- Mining and retrieving personal health information and opinions [127–130, 136],
- Measuring quality of document content or of healthcare interactions [49, 140],
- Analysing emotions and studying emotional effects [131, 135, 139],
- Determining clinical outcome [137],
- Detecting adverse drug events [134]

Mining and retrieving health information and opinions as well as determining clinical outcome are applications that are also relevant when doing sentiment analysis of clinical narratives. However, additional applications are possible. A few examples will be presented in the following.

Health Status Aggregation For physicians, sentiment analysis results can be used to **identify and summarize the health status** of a patient and its development over time in general or for specific medical conditions (see Fig. 10.2). By extracting and aggregating the attitudes and intentions expressed in clinical narratives from all the cooperating physicians an approximate real status from different medical perspectives can be illustrated based on the extracted opinions. Physicians recognize the status of the patient progressively through examinations, observations and discussions with others. Each step reflects one aspect of the patient status. Recovering the status information and personal perceptions of single health carers is necessary to reconstruct the entire status of the patient, since it provides the connection between treatment, and the transition of treatments as well as the outcomes.

To demonstrate that use case, consider a patient with a long term medical condition such as diabetes. From time to time additional medical conditions occur related to diabetes. Multiple physicians are involved in the treatment. However, the general practitioner receives clinical summaries from the other colleagues and needs to aggregate this information. Sentiment analysis methods could be applied to generate a curve plotting the health status per medical condition over time. Extended by events such as update of medication or dosage, operation, or other treatments, such diagram could provide at the first glance an overview what the current status is and about the development of health. In this way, decision making can consider the integrated patient status reconstructed from the **"wisdom of crowds" scattered in multiple clinical narratives**.

Similarly, such graph could support patients in monitoring their health. When such graph is generated from patient questionnaires or online diaries, information

Table 10.2 Summary of sentiment analysis work in the domain of medicine

Textual source	Paper	Task	Method	Level	Resource	Application
Blogs	Denecke [49]	Information content	Logistic regression	Document	SentiWordNet, UMLS	Quality of social media
Blogs	Xia et al. [128]	Polarity	Multinomial Naive Bayes classification	Topic	–	Patient opinion mining
Blogs	Sharif et al. [134]	Polarity	K-means clustering	Document	SentiWordNet	Detecting adverse drug events
Tweets	Sokolova et al. [130]	Polarity	Naive Bayes, decision trees, k-nearest neighbor, SVM	Document	–	Mining personal health information
Forums	Biyani et al. [131]	Polarity	Co-training algorithm	Document	Adapted SL, Wikipedia	Analysing emotional effects
Forums	Tanveer et al. [127]	Polarity	Naive Bayes, SVM, logistic regression	Sentence	SL	Categorization

(continued)

Table 10.2 (continued)

Textual source	Paper	Task	Method	Level	Resource	Application
Forums	Sokolova and Bobicev [135]	Emotion	Naive Bayes, k-nearest neighbor	Document	WordNet Affect	Studying sentiments in forums
Forums	Melzi et al. [136]	Emotion	SVM	Document	EmoLex[121]	Patient knowledge retrieval
Drug reviews	Na et al. [129]	Polarity	Rule-based linguistic	Aspect (overall opinion, effectiveness, side effects, condition, cost, dosage)	SentiWordNet, SL, UMLS	Drug opinion mining
Suicide notes	Pestian et al. [139]	Emotion	Supervised learning	Token and sentence	–	Emotion analysis
Questionnaires	Cambria et al. [140]	Emotion	Rule-based and clustering	Document	ConceptNet, WordNet Affect	Measuring healthcare quality
Questionnaires	Smith et al. [133]	Polarity	Naive Bayes, SVM	Document	–	Sentiment classification, determining relevance of discourse function
Biomedical literature	Niu et al. [137]	Outcome	SVM	Document	UMLS	Determining clinical outcome

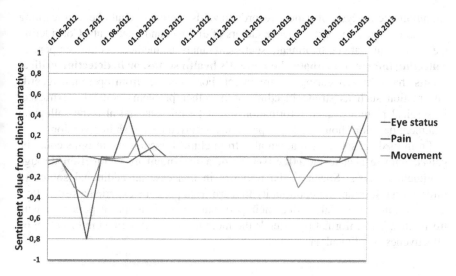

Fig. 10.2 Application of sentiment analysis to generate a health status graph. The graph shows the health status per single medical condition

can be compared to clinical information to see whether the clinical impression correlates with the patient's perceptions.

Quality Assessment For clinical decision making, but also from a quality management point of view, sentiment analysis could be used to **collect statistical information on the outcome of treatments** given some medical condition. Analyses are possible how often for example a complication or critical event occurred when some specific treatment was applied. Thus, for a hospital manager and resource planner, sentiment analysis results can provide a basic quantitative measurement based on different medical narratives which can be used as a reference for quality assessment, planning and scheduling.

Furthermore, consider a patient in palliative care (end-of-life-care): They require not only the anaesthetic treatment to eliminate the symptoms and pain, but also the mental support of the practitioners and the comfort from social connections. The feedback of the patient in the palliative ward is crucial to assess the effectiveness of the treatment. Based on the feedback from patients as it is reflected in nurse notes, different aspects of the treatment can be evaluated and further adjustment of the therapy can be conducted.

Outcome Research For researchers, sentiment analysis methods can be employed to extract and classify the outcome of medical treatments or learn about the effectiveness of treatments. Hence, the labour-intensive user studies for treatment can be facilitated. Furthermore, sentiment analysis could be exploited for performing a **retrospective analysis of treatment processes and outcome research**. Information about treatment outcome is captured in clinical documents and biomedical literature.

An automatic analysis of patient records towards sentiment could help in learning more about outcomes and influence factors of diseases and treatments. Considering the individual patient treatment, sentiment analysis methods could support in **collecting information about the patient's health status, or in detecting critical events** that occurred during the treatment. For example, from operation records information such as strong bleeding or on other problems could be extracted. In surgical planning, such information might be relevant and also the follow-up treatment decision should consider problems occurred during an intervention.

From medical social media, but also from clinical documents, insights could be gained with respect to the **effectiveness of a treatment or medication** through sentiment analysis. Social media provides in this case an additional source of information. It offers the opportunity to learn from patient's experiences since they are describing in social media, their personal perceptions and experiences with treatments. This information extends the more implicitly described information on effectiveness in clinical narratives.

10.4   Future Research Aspects of Sentiment Analysis in Medicine

In this section, research aspects to be considered in future are summarized that were derived from the analysis presented in Sect. 6.2.

10.4.1   Domain-Specific Sentiment Source

Through the word analysis, we recognized that terms such as *right, patient* are identified as polarity terms when applying general sentiment lexicons. This is due to the term ambiguity. In the medical context, these terms are used in an objective manner. Further, the sentiment lexicon SentiWordNet matched also many nouns which are labelled objective. The subjectivity lexicon (SL) originates from social media sources. It contains basic sentiment terms whereas SentiWordNet (SWN) was built on WordNet synsets. Its board coverage on terminology has already been proved by a larger recall in comparison to SL. In order to constitute a suitable lexicon with high precision for the medical domain, more context and domain knowledge should be considered to reduce the ambiguity during the matching process. Due to different language use, and the more objective way of writing in the clinical narratives, the conventional sentiment lexicons need to be adapted to cope with these peculiarities of medical narratives. Consider the word "positive". In clinical language, this term is often used contrarily to our normal usage. A "positive finding" has often negative implications to a patient (e.g. HIV test was positive means that the patient is infected with HIV). Further, the ambiguity and polysemy in the medical domain is different to the normal domain. Additionally, the implicit aspects of the polarity for medical terminology need to be considered (see Sect. 10.4.3).

The results showed that clinical documents do not contain the "classical" opinionated terms which are adjectives, but often nouns. In order to address this challenge, resources need to be developed, that link medical conditions with sentiment or their respective judgements. Such domain-specific resource could be created based on a basic medical ontology, enriched with polarity information and the corresponding inference approaches for concept dependency. Context could also be learned from training material.

10.4.2 Level of Analysis

Given the multiple notions of sentiment presented in Sect. 10.1, it becomes clear that the level of analysis needs to be carefully selected. In general, sentiments can be studied at document-, sentence- or topic-level. For sentiment analysis from clinical narratives, topic- or aspect-level sentiment analysis should be chosen. A clinical document summarizes many information on the health status of a patient; it can apparently not be related to one single topic. Authors of clinical documents express their attitudes and observations with respect to certain body parts or medical conditions of one patient at sentence level. Interpretation of sentiment and judgements in medical sentiment analysis requires also consideration of the context (which means sometimes looking beyond document boundaries). The particular challenge that goes beyond existing research on topic- or aspect-level sentiment analysis, is that a domain-specific knowledge base needs to be incorporated that supports in aggregating the aspects. For example, problems with a stomach might be described through multiple symptoms: *diarrhoea, abdominal pain, nausea.* Background knowledge is necessary, to recognize that these symptoms belong to the same medical condition.

Additionally, the sentiment categories need to be carefully selected depending on the sentiment notion under consideration. The concrete patient status implied by medical conditions cannot simply be judged as positive, negative or neutral. For example, the disease may be not deadly for the patient but can bring a lot of pain. Is that positive or negative? Some other disease may not cause any pain to the patient, but can be quite urgent and severe. In order to represent these situations, more detailed aspects should be given instead of conventional polarity (positive or negative). In particular, when we are considering medical conditions, aspects of sentiment are *presence, certainty* and *severity* (see Sect. 10.1). New categories of sentiment need to be specified.

10.4.3   Explicit and Implicit Sentiments

The clinical narratives differ from social media data in terms of word usage. That was confirmed by our analysis. In contrast to sentiments in non-medical social media, where opinion and polarity is manifested in corresponding words (mainly adjectives), in clinical narratives sentiment is often contained implicitly and needs to be inferred among others from the medical concepts used in documents. Implicit descriptions of the health status concern mentions of critical symptoms (e.g. *severe pain, extreme weight loss, high blood pressure*). An explicit description of the health status is reflected through phrases such as *the patient recovered well* or *normal*. In particular, the outcome of a treatment can often only be derived from the described effects of a treatment to a medical condition. For example, a statement that a medical condition improved allows to draw the conclusion that the treatment had a positive outcome. This impacts the necessary analysis methods. More knowledge-relevant and context-dependent features need to be chosen to cope with the characteristics of text in the medical domain.

10.4.4   Medical Sentiment Analysis: The Future

In summary, the following research challenges need to be addressed when analysing medical texts (medical social media text, clinical narratives) with respect to sentiment:

- Modelling of implicit clinical context and determining implicit sentiment,
- Building upon a domain-specific sentiment lexicon,
- Determining sentiment depending on the contexts, and
- Modelling different aspects of the patient status.

Additional aspects are determining the opinion holder and considering time. During the treatment, the health status is supposed to improve, but can also worsen. An operation could start normally, but can become critical. For this reason, medical sentiment should also be considered over time. Time is provided by document time stamps or sometimes in the documents themselves or clinical data could be sorted according to treatment phases. As other studies already showed, negations are used very frequently in clinical narratives. In sentiment analysis, it is crucial to identify negations since polarity can be reversed (e.g. in *no complaints of pain when asked*). Existing algorithms such as NegFinder [143] or NegEx [144] can be exploited for this purpose.

Part IV
Applications

Social media tools and web technologies can be simply used in healthcare settings. Recapture, that we mainly considered medical social media data, that provide a complementing resource for information gathering, treatment, or disease monitoring. So the question is how the methods presented in the previous chapters can be exploited and integrated to make use of this social media data space. In this part of the book, some example applications will be described. One essential application is the monitoring of public health through social media data. Health organizations can benefit from new surveillance capabilities. Second, retrieving relevant social media content would be beneficial for multiple users. A diversity-aware retrieval engine will be introduced that targets at providing diverse search results to improve user satisfaction.

Chapter 11
Social Media for Health Monitoring

For public security issues (e.g., monitoring terroristic activities), social media is already considered intensively. This matter is acknowledged also by the public health community [145]. In the last couple of years, public health authorities and epidemiologists became increasingly aware that it is no longer sufficient to consider indicator-based data from patient records or collected through active reporting for disease surveillance since the time delay is often immense. Thus, health authorities started to use additional information for the purpose of early warning and disease outbreak prevention. These developments were summarized by the term "Epidemic Intelligence" [146]. Epidemic Intelligence comprises an early identification, assessment and verification of potential public health hazards and a timely dissemination of alerts. It relies heavily on established indicator sources such as number of reported infections, drug prescriptions, etc.

For example, epidemiologists at the European Centre of Disease Prevention and Control (ECDC) use the MedISys system [147] to check local news for disease outbreak information. Scientific assessments of the utility of Web Mining for the domain of public health showed that it could help in overcoming time delays in reacting to health threats, among others by providing additional information about outbreaks [148].

MediSys and other news monitoring systems mainly present texts that are determined as relevant by the system and resist on aggregating information referring to the same health event into signals. Beyond online news, another frequently assessed source are search logs from search engines such as Google Flu Trends. Evaluations of those approaches concentrated so far on a comparison of the results with data from health statistics (indicator-based data). For example, several papers correlated the output of Google Flu Trends with influenza outbreak statistics [149–151].

In the remainder of this chapter, a concrete system, the M-Eco system, is described. It considers information from multiple sources and aggregates relevant

© Springer International Publishing Switzerland 2015
K. Denecke, *Health Web Science*, Health Information Science,
DOI 10.1007/978-3-319-20582-3_11

information into signals that are presented with various presentation options to a user. Parts of this section have been published as journal paper [36] by the book author in collaboration with members of the M-Eco project consortium.

11.1 M-Eco System

M-Eco exploits data from multiple sources for public health monitoring purposes. The system:

- Monitors social media, TV, radio and online news,
- Aggregates texts into signals,
- Visualizes the signals using geographic maps, time series and tag clouds,
- Allows searching and filtering signals along various criteria (location, time, medical condition).

In a nutshell, the system works as follows: Texts from social media and TV/radio are continuously collected. Social media sources comprise among others texts from Twitter, blogs, and fora. TV and radio transmissions are recorded via satellite and transcribed automatically to text. The transcripts are used as input to the system. In the following, the term "text" is used to refer to some piece of text which can be for example a tweet, a blog posting, or even a transcript of a TV or radio transmission. A text is annotated with linguistic information; disease names, persons and locations are identified and labelled with their semantic class. These features provide an input to machine learning algorithms that detect patterns in the data. The patterns are analysed and signals are generated automatically when unexpected behaviour is determined. A signal is a hint to some anomalous event. Since the amount of generated signals can overwhelm a user, recommendation techniques are exploited to filter out those signals that are of potential interest for a particular user. The information related to a signal is shown in charts and through personalized tag clouds to allow users to easily assess signals. To realize these steps, the M-Eco system consists of a set of web services that cover four areas depicted in Fig. 11.1. These are (1) content collection, (2) signal generation, (3) user modelling and recommendation as well as (4) visualization in a user interface. The services work in a pipeline fashion and are triggered automatically four times a day. The processing within the four components is described in more detail in the following paragraphs.

Recapturing the architecture for textanalytic-enabled systems introduced in Chap. 7, the M-Eco system consists of:

- A collection service (content collection component),
- An NLP service (document analysis component),
- Two filtering services (signal generation component and recommendation component),
- Two visualisation services (for timeline visualisation and tag cloud generation,

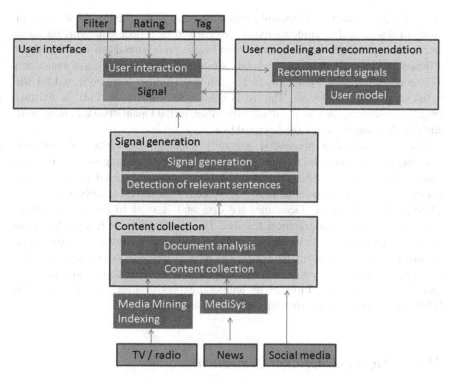

Fig. 11.1 Components and processing pipeline of the M-Eco system

- Several resources (social media sources to crawl, TV and radio channels to record, list with disease and symptom names, geographic coordinates, user preferences, training material).

11.1.1 Content Collection and Document Analysis Component

The information database of the system is filled continuously by the content collector and document analysis component. It collects data from various sources by means of web crawling and streaming APIs, and makes them accessible to other components. The collection focuses on broadcast news from TV and radio, news data from MedISys [147], and social media content from blogs, forums and Twitter. The TV and radio data is collected via satellite and transcribed to written text by SAIL's Media Mining Indexing System [152].

Blogs and forums are collected from their corresponding RSS feeds. A streaming API from Twitter allows downloading a subset of Twitter data containing keywords from a predefined list. About 1300 names of symptoms and diseases were used as keywords. These keywords were manually collected by epidemiologists as part of the M-Eco system development process, starting from a list of 18 diseases or group of diseases. The epidemiologists were asked to collect synonyms for these diseases, in particular terms used by non-health professionals to describe these diseases and related symptoms. In total, 386 terms referring to disease names and 872 terms referring to symptoms in English and German were collected for the initial version of the system. The list is continuously extended. Further, existing language resources such as WordNet, GermaNet, or the OpenOffice thesaurus were additionally used to extend the keyword lists.

The data collection process is generally language-dependent. All collected relevant texts are processed by a set of natural language processing tools. The data is tokenized and part-of-speech-tagged by the Tree Tagger and parsed by the Stanford Parser. All texts are also semantically annotated. Four different tools are applied: BURGeoN[1] is based on Geonames.org data and is used to annotate locations and to disambiguate geographical features. The identification of terms referring to symptoms and diseases is based on a pre-defined list of known entities (the same list that is used for collecting the texts). The recognition of those entities is realized as a minimal finite state automaton that was built for both, diseases and symptoms. HeidelTime [153] is used to identify temporal expressions and the Stanford NER [154] is used to detect information on affected organisms.

11.1.2   Signal Generation Component

The event detection and signal generation component exploits the annotated texts provided by the content collection and document analysis component to generate signals. It produces signals with associated information on the disease or symptom the signal is referring to and a location that has been extracted for that signal. In a first step, relevant sentences are separated from irrelevant ones using a transfer-based machine learning classifier based on support vector machines and considering the annotated information as features (sentence position, part-of-speech tag tree, named entities including disease names, location, person) [155].

The classifier is based on the open source implementation of the SVMTK by Moschitti [156]. The algorithm automatically classifies outbreak reports (from ProMed Mail [157] and WHO) to train a supervised learner. The knowledge acquired from the learning process is then transferred to the task of classifying social media texts. Our experiments showed that with the automatic classification of training data and the transfer approach, an overall precision of 92 % and an accuracy of 78.20 % is achieved (tested on blogs from the Avian Flu Diary [158]).

Sentences are classified as relevant or irrelevant by the method presented before. For all relevant sentences, entity pairs (location, disease) are exploited to produce time series. A time series is produced for each entity pair occurring in sentences of

---

[1] www.fit.vutbr.cz/~iotrusina/BURGeoN-0.1.tar.gz.

texts published within 1 week. The sentences determined as relevant are also made
available in the visualization for the user when assessing a signal. This helps to
concentrate on the relevant sentences during manual information analysis.

The time series provide then the input for statistical methods for signal generation, CUSUM and Farrington. These two statistical methods have originally
been developed for indicator-based surveillance [159]. Cumulative sum or CUSUM
methods originated in quality control [160]. They focus on several consecutive
periods, and sum up the aberrations in one particular direction. Farrington et al.
proposed an approach based on generalized linear models [161], which is by
now broadly applied in European countries for indicator based surveillance. The
Farrington approach fits a regression model to the data over several years, allowing
for a secular trend. Outbreaks in the past are automatically identified and removed,
and the statistical distribution fits either to rare counts or to frequent counts. The user
interface allows them to select signals from the one or the other algorithm. Between
zero and fifty signals are generated by this procedure every night. The exact number
depends on several variables or factors that influence the generation of signals such
as the type of considered data (e.g. Twitter's update frequency is much higher than
of a blog).

Further, the following properties of the signal generation algorithm need to be
considered:

1. In order to contribute to a signal, at least one entity referring to a disease or
   symptom, e.g. "measles", has to occur in a sentence (or the text it was taken
   from).
2. A signal is generated when the threshold for the number of associated sentences
   or texts containing the same disease entity is exceeded. The threshold is based
   on an empirical value, but at least two sentences or texts with the same keyword
   need to exist.
3. The sentences or texts that contribute to a signal must have to fall into the same
   time frame which is set to 1 day.

11.1.3 Recommendation Component

The recommendation component gets as input the generated signals and either
selects those that are of interest for a user according to his profile or ranks the signals
appropriately. The component also supports users with personalized presentation
options (e.g., tag clouds, list of recommendations) that are visualized in the user
interface. In this way, information or alerts are filtered before being presented to a
user which in turn reduces information overload. The recommendation component
requires a user profile that consists of information on user behaviour from interactions with the system (e.g., ratings, tags, search terms).

The personalization and recommendation of signals mainly relies upon the
tagging behaviour of a user. Tags are potential indicators of user preference.

For instance, a medical expert that has exhaustively assigned the tag "swine flu" to the texts he evaluates, seems to be interested in that disease. Therefore, this knowledge can be utilized to filter out irrelevant recommendations unrelated to "swine flu". For recommending items to the user, tags assigned by him to his texts of interest are compared against the tags assigned to candidate and unknown texts.

In order to help users navigating through a vast collection of texts and finding new items, a tag cloud component provides a visual representation of texts. Besides indexing texts in the corpus, each tag helps users to find new related information of interest. Tag clouds were chosen as the core retrieval interface for exploring specific texts. A subset of texts is retrieved by a clicking on the term available in the tag cloud. Terms called tags displayed in the tag cloud are defined by users or automatic annotation tools. Therefore, various combinations of tags result in different subsets of retrieved texts and all emerging trends and relationships in the available set of texts can be explored.

The tag cloud interface performs semantic and syntactic grouping to avoid tag redundancies in the tag cloud. Semantically similar tags are depicted with the same color and positioned nearby each other. For clustering tags into semantic groups, the K-means algorithm was exploited that considers each tag from a tag space as feature vector. By this clustering of tags, it is easier for a user to notice and discover relations and connections between depicted tags.

11.1.4   User Interface and Visualization

The user interface allows a user to search for disease names or symptoms and to assess the related signal information by means of a geographic map, a tag cloud or a timeline. The geographic map plots the signals to a map. It enables the user to select specifically signals related to locations that are interesting for him. The timeline shows the text volume referring to a specific disease or symptom (or the corresponding signal, respectively) over time.

This allows users to learn about the progress of a disease outbreak as reflected in social media and also about seasonal differences. The tag cloud provide a quick overview on the content of the texts associated with a signal. They enable the user to quickly decide about the relevance of a signal. Access to the original sources that contributed to the signal generation is provided as well as filtering capabilities (e.g. selecting a time span). Beyond, user feedback options were included into the user interface. With "Thumbs up - thumbs down" and a rating scale for signals, users can judge the relevancy of the presented signal. This information is fed back to the recommendation process and considered for ranking and filtering. Through those services described before, M-Eco offers (1) additional information through social media monitoring, (2) perception of recommendation and users behaviour and (3) visualization and support for risk assessment. Screenshots of the system are shown in Figs. 11.2 and 11.3.

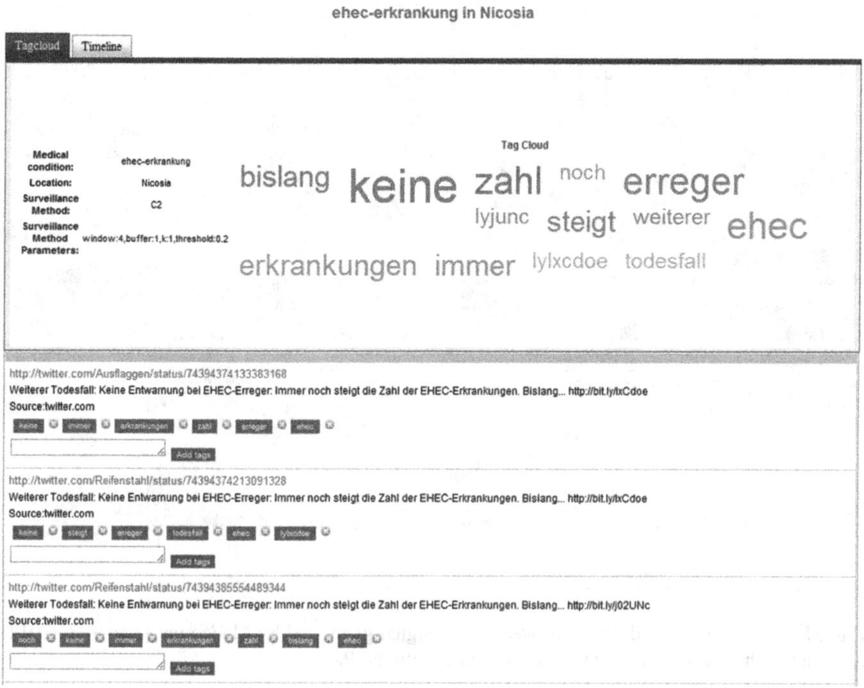

ehec-erkrankung in Nicosia

Fig. 11.2 Tag cloud view of texts from a selected signal

11.2 Experiences and Lessons Learnt

Contrasting the initial expectation, the signals were not generated from clustered reports on personally reported symptoms, but on news reports that were fed into social media, and replicated or forwarded by interested users. Therefore, M-Eco was not the first instance to detect the public health event, because there were local actors who had already detected and reported about the event. However, M-Eco brought such reports quickly to a broader attention.

Assessments of the M-Eco system results revealed characteristics of social media that are relevant for disease surveillance. First, the texts that contributed to signals rated as relevant by the epidemiologist often linked to media reports or so-called secondary reports. This experience let conclude that there might be a trend in social media whereby users tend to write less often about their personal specific symptoms, but most often forward information from reliable sources such as news sites, or preventions efforts from authorities.

Second, most signals were generated from Twitter data. The volume of relevant Twitter data that is processed by the system is much higher than from any other source considered as input. Beyond, the coverage of social media is still an open issue. It is unclear who is providing relevant health information via social media,

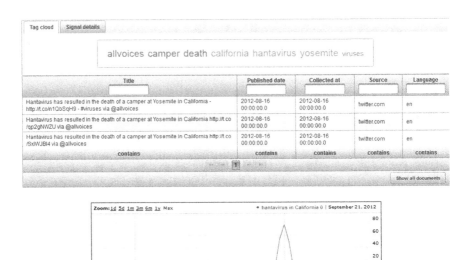

Fig. 11.3 Time series and detected tweets for a signal generated by M-Eco on August 16, 2012 referring to the Hantavirus outbreak at Yosemite National Park

which age groups, personal background of persons might play a role, geographic coverage etc. Another challenge is the quality of content collected from social media and the difficulty to automatically decide whether it is a real outbreak or not. Many of the social media texts present vague reports of illnesses. This means that technology is in principle ready for monitoring social-media data for disease surveillance purposes.

Chapter 12
Diversity-Aware Search

To support users in identifying relevant information in the medical web, on the one hand, standards for medical web content were defined to allow certification of quality health information (e.g. the HONcode certification[30]). However, such certificate does not help a user to assess the diverse aspects of web content. Therefore, on the other hand, users need support in finding relevant content by more sophisticated search facilities. Existing web and medical blog search engines (e.g., Medworm [162]) list search results matching query keywords in a flat list. Diversity is—if at all—only considered by presenting different results in the top N positions.

However, the content of a document in general, or of medical social media in particular, can be diverse due to the background of an author, the source (e.g., blog, forum), topic etc. For example, a text on *diabetes* can discuss not only symptoms, but also treatments, related diseases, and possible medications. Following this intuition, we consider a document to be diverse when it covers different aspects of a topic or when a topic is described in different ways (i.e., in a factual or affective manner).

In this chapter, a system architecture for a retrieval engine is introduced that allows to exploit (medical) domain specific notions of diversity [163]. We follow the assumption that more users are satisfied with a result set when texts are shown in the top N positions that are diverse in their aspects considered and their type of information content (factual vs. affective). Several usage scenarios for such retrieval engine are possible: A health professional needs diverse information since he might be interested in getting information on some rare diseases, but also in experiences from other physicians in treating patients with this disease. A diverse result set is crucial for a patient who can be interested in learning more about the disease he or she is suffering from, its treatments and medications, but also in experiences from other patients in living with the disease.

© Springer International Publishing Switzerland 2015
K. Denecke, *Health Web Science*, Health Information Science,
DOI 10.1007/978-3-319-20582-3_12

12.1   Diversity in Web Search and Medical Social Media

Research on information retrieval in the biomedical domain has focused on the retrieval of biomedical research publications [164–166]. These highly specialised text mining applications incorporate natural language processing capabilities, particularly specialised for the biomedical domain, complex algorithms and rules based on scientific vocabularies [167]. Research in that area has focused on improving search results by taking domain knowledge into account [168]. To reduce an overload of low-quality pages in search results, specialised search engines have been set up including Curbside.md for physicians or Healthline for patients. These search engines only retrieve content from professional sources or at least from verified sources.

Several studies have shown that users usually prefer diversified search results [169–171], i.e. results that are dissimilar. Thus, diversity is introduced as measure for dissimilarity. Result diversification is realised by finding the best trade off between diversity and similarity [172]. It targets finding the right balance between having more relevant results of the "correct" intent and having more diverse results in the top positions [173, 174]. However, the notions of diversity that have been taken into account so far are still restricted to certain kinds of general content or category similarity, though a large range of more specific types of diversity exist [175].

Besides classical search engines that provide flat lists of search results and that consider diversity only in the ranking of results, there exist faceted search that allows to explore a search result by filtering along some facets [176]. Such systems assign multiple classes to one object which allows ordering in multiple ways [177]. The classes capture the different facets, i.e., dimensions or features, relevant to a collection. Diederich and Balke considered faceted search as an alternative for keyword search for biomedical literature [178]. However, their facet analysis methods group text only according to topics. Additional dimensions of diversity remain unconsidered. Similarly, the French portal CISMeF (Catalog and Index of French-speaking Health Resources [179]) allows to filter search results along two dimensions: document type (recommendations and guidelines, pedagogical resources, documents concerning patients) and target audience (professionals. students, patients). Diversity is provided at the result set level.

Hliaoutakis et al. introduce MedSearch [180], a specialised search engine for medical information that provides diversified search results. For result diversification, web pages are clustered together when they describe the same topic. In the ranking, each cluster contributes at most one page.

12.2 Diversity Dimensions: Information Type and Aspects Considered

The approach presented in the following looks at the content of social media documents and thus, considers diversity on document- or content-level. Two diversity dimensions related to the content of a document are analysed with domain specific features of the medical domain and considered for ranking. The two dimensions are *aspects considered* and *type of information content*. To explain these two notions consider the following example: Assuming that there is a blog written by a patient suffering from depression. In some of her posts, she is writing about her daily life, i.e. about experiencing depression, feeling lost and sad. She is providing her experiences in living with that disease. In other postings she presents information on the medical treatments, diagnostic aspects and medications related to this disease. The type of information content of the single posts differs, changing between information and experience. Further, the postings consider different aspects of the disease, which are aspects of the diagnosis, treatment or medication. In general, we would assume that these two dimensions of diversity are independent from each other. However, it might be that some aspects are discussed rather from a personal view point than others. Future work needs to assess whether these dimensions are orthogonal or whether there are dependencies between aspects considered and the type of information content.

We can distinguish two categories of information content: factual and affective. They occur due to varying author intents. Correspondingly, two measures can be defined to quantify the type of information content, $degree_{fac}$, and $degree_{aff}$. The diversity of aspects considered is seen as the variety in medical concepts or their semantic categories, respectively. As medical concepts we consider concepts that are contained in biomedical vocabularies or ontologies such as the Unified Medical Language System. The semantic types and main groups are exploited for measuring the diversity of some input text. Two measures are used to describe the diversity of aspect considered, div_{type}, and div_{group}. The calculation of the diversity measures is described in the following section.

12.3 Architecture for Diversity-Aware Search in Medical Social Media

Briefly, the system works as follows: From a set of relevant online sources new content is collected regularly. The diversity of the single texts is assessed by calculating diversity measures. Given a search query provided by a user, the system retrieves medical blogs and other social media content matching the query from the previously collected and indexed data. The diversity measures are exploited when the result set is ranked and presented to the user.

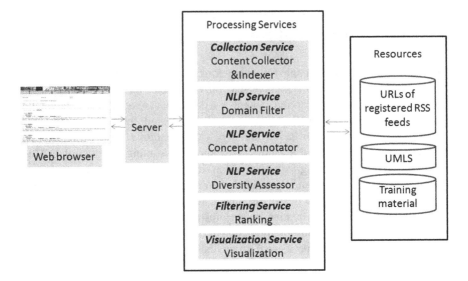

Fig. 12.1 Architecture of the retrieval engine: Processing services are coordinated by a server and make use of knowledge resources

The diversity-aware retrieval engine is implemented as a service-oriented architecture (see Fig. 12.1) and implements the framework for textanalytic-enabled systems introduced in Chap. 7. The search interface allows the user to interact with the system. The server is responsible for triggering services in the correct order and for the communication between user interface and services. We can distinguish four types of services:

- Collection service: Content collector and indexer
- NLP services: Domain filter, concept annotator, diversity assessor
- Filtering service: Ranking
- Visualization service: Visualization

Several resources are used by the system including the UMLS, a list of URLs of relevant sources and training material for the algorithms. The components are described in more detail in the following.

12.3.1   Content Collector and Indexer

The content collector crawls RSS feeds for registered blogs every day and collects the corresponding postings. HTML tags are removed and the actual text is stored in a database from which a Lucene index is built. This index is queried when a user enters a query to the system to find information.

Blogs that should be considered for collection are manually identified and registered to the system. As shown in previous work [181], the strategy of manually selecting sources for crawling is useful (and often necessary) to reduce the noise introduced to the search results when considering web pages or blogs without filtering. Therefore, we decided to manually register the blogs from which content is collected. This procedure intends to ensure a certain quality of content. At the same time, users are enabled by this to build an engine that is specific to their needs since they can add or remove sources to be considered by the search engine. To receive a sufficient number of retrieval results, the more blogs are registered the better. Another influence factor is the update frequency of blogs: When a blog is only updated once a month, substantially more blogs need to be considered by the content collector to get a sufficient number of texts.

12.3.2   Domain Filter

Even in blogs that are known for dealing with medical and health issues, postings that do not contain medical content may appear. These postings are filtered out by a domain filter. The Alchemy categorizer [182] is used for this purpose. It assigns the most likely category to a text based on statistical algorithms and natural language processing technology. Texts to which Alchemy assigns a category other than the category *health* are excluded from further processing.

12.3.3   Concept Annotator

In a next step, medical entities are extracted from relevant texts by an ontology-based biomedical text annotation tool provided by the Dragon Toolkit [62]. This tool uses an approximate dictionary lookup to extract terms that refer to concepts of the UMLS. From the resulting set of concepts, the number of different semantic groups and main categories is determined using the concept information. Further, the number of concepts describing diseases, medical treatments and medications is calculated, by counting concepts belonging to the main categories *disorder, procedure* or *chemical and drugs*.

12.3.4   Diversity Assessor

The diversity assessor analyses the collected content with respect to the *aspects considered* and the diversity of *information content*. It exploits the number of semantic types and main categories determined by the concept annotator for calculating the diversity measures: div_{type}, div_{group}, $degree_{fac}$, and $degree_{aff}$. A high diversity in *aspect considered* is reflected by a large variety in semantic types or main groups. This is considered in formulae (1) and (2) that calculate the proportion of different semantic types (main groups) contained in a text to measure diversity. A value close to 1 indicates a high diversity, while a value close to 0 corresponds to a small diversity. The number "135" refers to the semantic types provided by the UMLS, while "15" is the number of UMLS semantic groups.

- $div_{type} = \frac{types}{135}$
- $div_{group} = \frac{groups}{15}$

Further, the diversity of *information content* is determined. In general, factual texts can be distinguished from affective texts. To describe the type of information content more precisely, the degree of factual or affective content is calculated by:

- $degree_{fac} = \frac{c}{words}$
- $degree_{aff} = \frac{o}{words}$

with c as the number of extracted medical concepts of a document d and o as the number of opinionated words in d, and words as the number of words in d. For the number of extracted medical concepts, only concepts describing disorders, procedures and medications are considered relevant. This decision was made since we had in mind users that search for such information. It is clearly possible to broaden the scope of the retrieval engine and consider also other UMLS categories when determining the medical content of a text.

Additionally, this service distinguishes *factual* from *affective* postings. Affective parts of a text are reflected by opinionated words. To count the opinionated words in a text, words that are neither medical content nor stop words can be looked up in SentiWordNet [183]. The measures $degree_{fac}$ and $degree_{aff}$ are exploited together with the number of words and the number of stop words as input for a supervised machine learning algorithm. Through experiments with different machine learning algorithms implemented in the WEKA library [184], the SimpleLogistic classifier [185] has been chosen since it outperformed Naive Bayes and other algorithms. The algorithm performed with 86.5 % accuracy in tenfold cross validations on 750 factual and 750 affective blog postings. This text material has been classified manually and also provides the training material within the diversity assessor.

12.3.5 *Ranking*

The results matching a query are ranked considering the diversity measures div_{type} and div_{group} as boosting factors. The main assumption is that postings with a larger diversity in types and groups are of higher interest to the user than those with a smaller diversity. In our experiments, this assumption will be studied.

12.3.6   Visualization

The user interface presents the ranked results. It consists of a single line text field for the query and a result section. Factual and affective texts can be shown separately. In addition, per1centages are listed for the categories disease, treatment and medication. They show to what extent a posting considers the single aspects and thus allow to quickly judge upon the general theme of a posting with respect to a query.

12.4   User Satisfaction with Diverse Retrieval Engine: Experiments

In this section, we summarise an experiment performed to study the user satisfaction with retrieval results when applying the introduced approach.

12.4.1   Data Set

As data set, the MSM data set was used (see Sect. 3.3). Five hundred and seventy-four of the collected postings were classified as affective, 12,299 were labeled factual by the classifier. The diversity of main group varies between 0.6 and 0.07 with an average value of 0.36. The average value for the diversity of semantic type was much lower with 0.157 (maximum: 0.52, minimum: 0.01) which results in a small diversity with respect to semantic types.

12.4.2   Evaluation Objectives and Setup

For the user evaluation, thirty queries were selected from studies on health-related web searches (see Table 12.1, [186]). These queries were chosen since they have been determined as frequently occurring queries in web search—at least for health professionals. The average query length was 2.6 words per query. For each query, the top 5 posts collected by a standard Lucene search engine with a scoring function were collected. Top 5 was chosen since other research showed that "few users look at results below the top 5" [187].

Our evaluation objective is to study the user satisfaction with an adapted ranking that considers the diversity measures. A scoring function is applied to the result list and is exploited to re-rank the results retrieved for a specific query. It considers the

Table 12.1 Queries used for retrieval selected from [189]

Query	No.	Query	No.
Oral hygiene, dental hygiene	9	Computerized patient record, CPR	6
Diabetes insulin pump	27	Colorectal cancer	60
Weight loss	319	Ultrasound	108
Vaccination	286	Multiple sclerosis	86
Surgery	769	Bacteria	202
Pancreas	45	Prevention breast cancer, screening breast cancer, screening mammography	90
Diabetic foot	9	Screening prostate cancer, prevention prostate cancer	46
Liver	707	Heart	1000
Sickle cell anemia	9	Injection	163
Anesthesia	31	Diabetes mellitus, diabetic diet, diet therapy, diet counseling, diet education	10
Obesity, health promotion diet, nutrition	438	Autonomic nervous system	4
Abortion	33	Asthma	302
Child abuse	58	Bronchitis, bronchiolitis bronchi	19
Low back pain	118	Chest pain, angina pectoris	97
HIV	485	Pain	1000

Each cell in the table contains one query. The number indicates the number of documents retrieved from our data set

diversity measures to get several rankings (or orderings) of the results. The scoring function is modified by a boost factor b which is multiplied into the TFxIDF score of hits. Six different rankings are determined, namely rankings with a TFxIDF based scoring function

- without boost factor, i.e. b = 1,
- with a boost factor b = 2 for documents classified affective,
- with a boost factor b = 2 for documents classified factual,
- with the value for group diversity as boost factor, i.e. $b = div_{group}$,
- with the value for type diversity as boost factor b, i.e. $b = div_{type}$,
- with the product of diversity measures as boost factor, i.e. $b = div_{group} * div_{type}$.

In the experiments, ten users had to rate the result sets with respect to relevancy as (0) irrelevant, (1) relevant, (2) highly relevant to the given query. The users were students of medical informatics. To create the evaluation result set to be assessed by the users, for each query the matching texts were retrieved from the data set. For this result set, we produced six different orderings by applying the scoring function with the six different values for the boost factor introduced before. From these orderings, we kept the top 5 results for each boost factor. The items included in the top 5 were the same for the six rankings per query, but they differed in the ordering.

Each user had to assess about 149 documents for all thirty queries, being neither aware of the ranking algorithm, nor of the ranking of each assessed post. The ranking results of the engines are compared based on user assigned ratings. The quality of each ranking was assessed using the normalized version of discounted cumulative gain (NDCG [188]). Discounted cumulative gain (DCG) is used in information retrieval to measure the effectiveness of a web search engine algorithm. Using a graded relevance scale of documents in a search engine result set, DCG measures the usefulness, or gain, of a document based on its position in the result list. The gain is accumulated from the top of the result list to the bottom with the gain of each result discounted at lower ranks. Problems with DCG occur when evaluations need to be compared and also when it should be assessed how good a retrieval engine really is: A low DCG value does not necessarily mean that the retrieval system is performing badly (maybe there are no good matches). For this purpose, the NDCG is used for comparing different lists of recommendations with various lengths. It is computed by dividing the DCG by the Ideal Discounted Cumulative Gain or IDCG. The IDCG is calculated similar to the DCG, but from a result list that is ordered by relevance. The higher the NDCG, the better is the ranked list. An average NDCG value was calculated over all queries and users. All results of the evaluation were tested for statistical significance using T-tests.

12.4.3 Results

The best value of 0.98 for NDCG has been calculated for the adapted scoring function where the boost factor is the product of diversity of group and type (Table 12.2). This average NDCG value is with a confidence of 99 % significantly higher than the value for ranking function *noboost* (NDCG value of 0.9). The average NDCG value for the adapted scoring function where affective texts are boosted (see ranking 2) is with 0.91 only slightly higher than the value for *noboost*. The same holds true for the ranking 3 where factual texts are ranked higher. The difference of NCDG values is not statistically significant for these two rankings. Since the top 5 results were the same for all boost factors per query and differed only in the ordering, the higher NDCG must have its origin in the different ranking.

Table 12.2 Values for NDCG for the rankings with different boost factors

Ranking	NDCG
1. No boost	0.909
2. Boost affective	0.910
3. Boost factual	0.909
4. Boost div_{group}	0.961
5. Boost div_{type}	0.965
6. Boost $div_{group} * div_{type}$	0.982

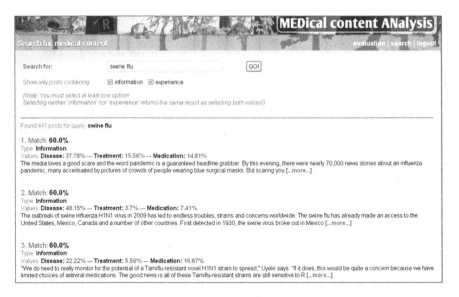

Fig. 12.2 Retrieval result interface: For each result item, the information type is shown (factual/affective). Further, it shows to what extent the content of the result page falls into the three medical categories

We conclude that the diversity of information type does not improve the ranking very much. For this reason, our retrieval engine uses this information for presenting and filtering search results (see Fig. 12.2). Further, it can be stated that the introduced measures for diversity are worth considering in ranking. Even if only one of the two diversity measures are exploited as boost factors (ranking 4 and 5), the average NDCG value is higher than the unboosted ranking with a confidence of 95 %.

12.5   Diversity in Medical Social Media: Lessons Learnt

Retrieving relevant texts from the medical social media data space is essential for making this resource useful for knowledge gathering and analysis. In the presented system, diversity measures that consider medical concepts mentioned in a text and their categories are used to rank retrieval results. The evaluation results suggest that the diversity measure reflecting diversity of aspects considered are well suited for supporting ranking. It could be shown that users are satisfied with a result set when diverse texts are shown in the top N positions. Our assumption that we can increase user satisfaction by ranking texts that have a higher diversity in higher positions has been proven correct. A basic assumption of the whole approach is that users are interested in highly diverse content. Users, who are interested in extremely specialised information, remain so far unconsidered in our approach and will probably be unsatisfied. Further, the diversity measures considered here, help only to rank documents higher that are diverse with respect to diagnoses, treatments and medications. Giving the user the opportunity to select diversity measures to be considered or to define what diversity for him means could help to address this shortcoming.

The content collector in this work relies upon a set of manually registered blogs. This strategy was chosen to ensure a certain quality of the retrieved content. However, this procedure results already in a pre-filtering of content. Alternatively, web crawling techniques as provided via Spinn3R could be exploited to collect all medical related content in the web.

The described approach to diversity aware ranking (and retrieval) has been proven successful in improving user satisfaction. However, our evaluation is limited in a way that user satisfaction is expressed by retrieval effectiveness. Other aspects that influence user satisfaction such as the result presentation were not explicitly considered by the evaluation setup. The users provided the feedback that some postings they had to judge were only advertisements with medical keywords. The filtering algorithms need to be adapted to filter out such non-sense postings in advance. In the experimental data set the number of postings labelled *affective* was much smaller than the number of factual postings which might be the reason why considering the measures for the type of information content in ranking has not proven successful. In future, we will reconsider this ranking with a more balanced data collection to see whether this information can support ranking as well. However, users reported that filtering either factual or affective texts provides additional guiding for distinguishing reliable or less reliable information. Thus, at least for result presentation, the type of information content can be useful.

Domain filters and information extraction tools are still far from perfect. When the domain filter fails, it might have no influence to the introduced ranking since no medical information will be extracted. In that case, the diversity measures will be zero or close to zero. In case the concept annotator misinterprets terms and maps them to medical concepts, the ranking quality can suffer. Texts will then be ranked in higher positions even if their medical content is not diverse. Thus, for the performance of the introduced ranking it is crucial that the information extraction from medical social media texts performs well. The service-oriented design of the architecture allows exchanging and adding services easily. In this way, other UMLS mapping tools can be tested whose mapping procedures are probably better suited for social media data. So far, available mapping tools have been specialised on processing biomedical literature (e.g., NCBO Open Biomedical Annotator [189]) where the language is easier to analyse since often standard biomedical terminology is used. In contrast in social media texts, common language needs to be processed.

Part V
Influence Factors

Exploiting social media data in general and medical social media data in particular has huge potentials as it was shown in the previous chapters of that book. However, there are associated risks with respect to privacy, security and abuse of data. Politics and individuals are becoming more and more aware of those risks which led already to breakups of projects in domains outside the healthcare domain. For example, researchers from Hasso Plattner Institute collaborated in 2012 with the German Schufa Holding AG, a protection company for general creditworthiness. In a project, they wanted to exploit data from social networks to make predictions on the payment behaviour of individuals (SCHUFALab@HPI [190]). The project was stopped due to serious concerns of monitoring financial behaviour and conclusions that might be drawn from social media data with respect to creditworthiness. Thus, the question arises whether the exploitation of social media data is desired by the society and what needs to be considered to avoid abuse of the data. Are human rights violated through this usage?

In this section, factors will be discussed that are necessary to be considered when exploiting social media tools for healthcare purposes or analysing medical social media data. They comprise ethical and legal issues as well as organisational issues. Clearly, we can only sketch the main difficulties to make the reader aware of them and to consider them carefully when developing healthcare applications that exploit social media.

Chapter 13
Implementation Obstacles

13.1 A Broad Range of Challenges

When implementing social media data or tools into healthcare processes, several challenges need to be addressed. They reach from technical, functional, and formal issues to organizational challenges (e.g. integration into clinical workflows). Technical issues comprise among others:

- Privacy and security aspects,
- Trust (technical, systemic, interpersonal),
- Access rights,
- Data storage,
- Integration with data from clinical information systems (e.g. electronic health records).

When social-media tools are exploited to support the treatment process, it needs to be ensured that—in case patient data is exchanged through such tools—privacy and security issues are considered. This includes among others assigning access rights for the various persons that are involved in the process and might access the data. Within the context of applications supporting the treatment process, integration with clinical information systems would be crucial for the health carers. To realize this, we will discuss in Chap. 15 a concept for integrating clinical data with medical social media data by using digital patient models.

There are also formal requirements to be considered when exploiting social media tools and data in healthcare. They comprise among others:

- Ethical and legal issues,
- Quality of content, reliability of content, and
- Payment models.

Ethical and legal issues will be discussed in more detail in Sect. 13.2 and Chap. 14, respectively. Mainly in the context of information gathering from

© Springer International Publishing Switzerland 2015
K. Denecke, *Health Web Science*, Health Information Science,
DOI 10.1007/978-3-319-20582-3_13

the Internet and social media, ensuring information quality is crucial. To support users in identifying relevant information in the medical web, standards for web content were already defined to allow certification of quality health information (e.g. the HONcode certification (http://www.hon.ch)).

The participatory aspect of social media is its strength, but also a big challenge. Inaccurate information can be distributed through social-media channels and have related implications regarding patient health and safety. Reaching populations with lower socio-economic status might be a challenge as well. People often use social media platforms to share information that is very difficult to get from other sources or is not present. In combination with different sources of health information, including data from the electronic health record, social media may contribute to better understand the new health scenarios we are facing in personalised medicine, patient-specific treatment or pharmacovigilance. However, relying only upon social media is insufficient. It can provide additional information, but confirmation by means of official health data is crucial.

It is crucial to make clear to all involved parties that the consideration of social media in the healthcare treatment process should not replace any face-to-face visits, but could enable a close monitoring by giving the patient the chance for self-managing his disease, taking over responsibility and on the other hand, enable physicians to monitor the health status more closely. Thus, the tools need to be integrated in existing workflows and will also require adaptation of workflows. However, this workflow integration is important to foster the acceptance of the tools and active participation of involved stakeholders. We suggest to use the concept of digital patient modelling and model-based decision support for combining both data sources in clinical practice (see Chap. 15).

In this context, also payment models need to be established in order to implement social media usage into the treatment process. The working time a physician spends in monitoring and interacting with his patients through social-media tools need to be reimbursed accordingly. This is crucial to successfully include such tools into the treatment process. Ethical and legal issues are related to the usage of data posted through social-media tools. Such questions mainly arise in the context of applications for monitoring and analysing the data posted in social media. In this context, it is also important to clarify responsibilities. Imagine a health status monitoring tool exploited by a health organization identifies a group of sick persons based on their social-media chatter. In which manner should the health organization react? Are they allowed to react? These and similar questions need to be answered before such applications go online.

13.2 Legal Issues

Health data are highly sensitive. Not only do they contain information about the health status of individuals, but also comprise the information that allow to reveal the identity of a patient. In the EU, the use of personal data is governed by the

Directive 95/46/EC on the protection of individuals with regard to the processing of personal data. However, the directive only states general rules for processing personal data that are not directly applicable to individuals. One of the principles of the directive with respect to processing personal data is that the purpose for which data is collected and processed must be explicitly specified and the data can only be stored for the time of the study. The use of the data needs to be transparent to allow patients to give their consent. Personal data is defined as "any [data] relating to an identified or identifiable natural person" [191]. Several concepts, techniques, mechanisms and tools have evolved over the years for crucial aspects of data security [191]:

- Confidentiality: only authorised users are allowed to view the data,
- Integrity: only authorised users are allowed to modify the data,
- Availability: authorised users should be able to access the data,
- Authenticity: process of verifying a claimed identity e.g. by a user name and password pair,
- Accountability: ability to trace users who were responsible for performing a particular task on the data.

Medical social media data is clearly personal data. Blog users often provide their names or other information that allows to draw conclusions on their identity. Applying mechanisms for data security to medical social media data can become difficult. Confidentiality is not given when a patient is posting in a public forum. The host of blogs and forums has always the means to remove entries of an individual from the blog or forum. Users normally agree to this by accepting the conditions of use when registering for a blog or forum. Normally, users need to log into the forum to post to a forum of blog. Thus, authenticity is given. There are several questions with respect to these legal directives and the use of medical social media data: The data is stored anyway by the host—does this allow researchers to simply use the data? How to inform social media users about the use of the data when researchers are crawling? These and similar questions go hand in hand with ethical issues related to Health Web Science. They are discussed in the next chapter.

Chapter 14
Ethics in Health Web Science

In this section, we summarize and discuss the ethical implications of the aforementioned trends and applications of using medical social media data in healthcare settings and collect implications towards the implementation to be further addressed in the future. *Ethics* concerns two basic practical problems of human life: (1) What is worth seeking—that is, what goals of life are good? and (2) What individuals are responsible for—that is, what duties should they recognize and attempt to fulfil [192]? *Public health ethics* deals with the specific moral questions regarding public actions for disease prevention, life elongation, or psychological and physical well-being. This is in contrast to *medical ethics* which concentrates on the relationship between patients and doctors. The issue of how ethical principles may be applied to Health Web Science is a current challenge for researchers, but also for health professionals and patients alike.

The web is usually considered a public space and processing public data does not necessarily require informed consent. However, there are open-access forums, blogs etc. and non-public forums. Thus, when analysing web communication in general or in the healthcare context in particular, ethical concerns include [193]:

- Privacy,
- Intellectual property rights,
- Informed consent,
- Trust, and
- Authenticity.

Starting from the ethical challenges around big data and internet research, we collect in the following specific ethical issues in the healthcare setting to conclude finally with the implications for implementing medical social media applications and Health Web Science.

© Springer International Publishing Switzerland 2015
K. Denecke, *Health Web Science*, Health Information Science,
DOI 10.1007/978-3-319-20582-3_14

Results summarized in this chapter result from a review of literature (both white and grey) to collect ethical issues related to social media usage in healthcare and associated to big data and internet-based research combined with an environmental scan of popular and current applications and services in this area.

Further, feedback from members of the International Medical Informatics Association (IMIA) Social Media Working group [194] was collected through an E-mail discussion. This working group aims to be IMIA's vehicle for stakeholder engagement in social media and targets at identifying, exploring, collaborating, and disseminating research on the use of social media for healthcare. Its members comprise representatives of the international health informatics community. Within the group, applications of social media are explored with particular applications to: (1) health care delivery, (2) health care professional education, (3) public health, (4) clinical and disaster medicine and (5) research.

14.1 Ethics in the Big Data Era

Availability of big data or social media data changes the possibilities of what to do with the user data. The data can be de-anonymised, analysed and interpreted in multiple ways. A problem is that collection of social media data on users reached already a new dimension. It is almost impossible to judge the possibilities of big data analytics for an individual. By analysing what people are saying in the web, what they are buying, companies already predict what people might be interested in. What will the future be? Technology is already able to predict a range of highly sensitive personal attributes such as sexual orientation, happiness, addictive substances etc. from easily accessible digital records of behaviour [195]. Can we analyse people's chatter in the web, their online behaviour and predict the diseases they will suffer from?

There are the following facts to be considered when talking about ethics in Web Science:

- Social media data have been found to be highly predictive.
- The data collected can be compiled and analysed to determine correlations, predict behaviour or other issues. Technology can provide greater institutional analysis than was conceivable in previous years.
- Data on usage behaviour are collected automatically by various technology-based web tools or by web-based statistics. Internet users are largely unaware that the online tools are collecting data and which data is collected. They are further unaware, that the written texts they contribute is analysed and interpreted.
- Over time, additional data sources will become available for more sophisticated analysis.

It is a matter of fact that in the web, data on individuals is stored. Although nick names are used, often individuals could be identified. Another problem is that big data or internet-based research offers the possibility to "spy" indirectly. Researchers are analysing data from persons and draw conclusions from it that can under certain circumstances harm the person when made public. So the question is also: How to deal with the data? The unpredictable possibilities of big data analytics make it impossible to ask users for informed consent. Agreeing to an analysis today, we won't know what will be possible in the future.

One of the central ethical issues around big data is to distinguish "public" and "private" since this distinction implies whether or not informed consent is required. Can we consider an online communication private when it is visible without restriction to the public? Publication on the internet may have parallels with publishing a letter in a newspaper. However, people posting data online cannot always be assumed to be seeking "public visibility" [196]. A problem is that not all web users are completely aware of the consequences of posting information to the web. Eysenbach and Till state that the perception of privacy very much depends on a particular group's protocols and privacy boundaries, target audience and aims [196].

Society raises concerns regarding privacy issues in conducting research with social media data or even developing applications that analyse such data or exploit the social media tools. Given these privacy concerns, questions about the appropriateness of researchers' use of medical social media to collect information or contact participants or to monitor the health status requires attention.

While not exhaustive, the following list exemplifies the types of questions researchers must address when using big data:

- Does the forum or blog provider let users know that their behaviour and texts are being tracked and analysed?
- What and how much information should be provided to the users with respect to the research or study purpose?
- In which detail the analytical results are going to be published?
- How should researchers react to the data and analysis results?
- What obligations does a researcher have to inform about research results and who is the owner of the data?

Answers to these questions may differ from research question to another and needs to be carefully discussed and addressed when doing internet research, in particular in the healthcare domain, but also beyond.

14.2 Ethical Issues of Social Media in Healthcare

After raising ethical questions regarding internet research in general, we are now focusing on the specific issues of social media data analysis and processing in the healthcare domain. In particular, we discuss issues related to medical social media research and questions regarding the patient-doctor relationship that gets influenced by availability of medical social media data.

14.2.1   Ethical Issues in Medical Social Media Research

Conducting research on social media sites requires deliberate attention to consent, confidentiality, and security. Usually in health research, the researcher decides both, what will be asked and how, and participants choose whether and how to answer the questions. A similar approach can be used in the context of internet research in healthcare: researcher could post questions and people decide how and if to answer them before starting with the study. With respect to ethical issues, this approach is simple since people can be informed beforehand about how their replies will be used before they post them. According to Bond et al. [197], medical web researchers should

- consider whether an online social networking site is an appropriate place to implement a research study,
- offer opportunities to review informed consent documents at multiple times and in multiple locations throughout the study; and
- collect data outside the social networking site and store it behind secure firewalls to ensure it will not be accessible to any person on the social networking site.

However, more often, the texts that people have already posted are used in Health Web Science research. Whether this sort of research should be considered within a "human subjects" framework or a more general humanities framework has been debated for over 10 years [196].

Two studies collected and analysed the views of social media users regarding (unintended) participation in internet research. Moreno et al. [198] report a study to explore participants reactions to direct experience with Facebook research methods. The purpose of this study was to determine older adolescents responses after learning that they were participants in a research study that involved identification of participants using Facebook. User views on privacy issues related to conducting research with online social network data of users were collected. The authors report that the majority of the participants viewed the use of Facebook in a research study positively.

One reason for the positive attitude may be that participants do not perceive personal risks to disclosing large amounts of information. To address the concerns of persons with negative attitude towards their participation, it is suggested to promote a greater understanding of information sharing in a research setting [198].

Bond et al. [197] described an ethics case study of using Facebook to deliver a sexual education program to youth and young adults, with a focus on a description of potential ethical risks related to beneficence, information and comprehension, equity and special populations, and confidentiality and security. They explored the views of contributors to online diabetes discussion boards with regards to if (and how) they feel their contributions to boards should be used by health researchers [197]. To study this question, they performed an email interview. The participants agreed that forum posts are in the public domain and that aggregated information could be freely used by researchers. Using aggregated data is acceptable to the community that created it. Using quotations ranges from being totally acceptable to totally unacceptable. The qualitative research norm of using quotes to support findings is particularly challenging when trying to preserve anonymity when citing from medical social media data. The problem is that social media quotes (and their authors) can be easily retrieved using standard web search engines. This means that even anonymised citation would be in vain. A suggestion is to aggregate multiple quotes into a single aggregated quote that captures the essence of the original quotes.

Different types of online interactions also may require different approaches. People writing blogs and using their own names, promoted through media such as Twitter, might be more concerned with being cited whilst people writing under a pseudonym on a discussion board might be more concerned with anonymity. The Association of Internet Researchers agrees the concept of the human research subject is not a good fit with much online research, preferring to focus on practical issues such as harm, vulnerability and identification. Online data is a new type of data for health researchers. Rather than interviewees answering the researchers questions, the "participants" have put their views "out there" for researchers to find. This not only needs a new approach to research ethics, it also requires a new approach to research methods. The details of these identified issues still need to be debated amongst all stakeholders.

14.2.2   Social Media and the Patient-Doctor Relationship

In this section, we will look at the implications of social-media usage in traditional care settings, which involves patient-physician communication. Patient-physician communication in the traditional sense comprises the direct contact and questioning of the patient by the physician and the discussion of treatment options. Information on diseases, therapies, and medications is exchanged; sometimes administrative issues are clarified, such as making appointments. This communication is strongly characterized by medical confidentiality, trust, and privacy. Data is expected to be safely stored in the patient record, inaccessible to others, and even protected by law. With the development of web technologies, communication and monitoring in healthcare is starting to be outsourced to social media. Appointments can be made online, health information and even examination results can be distributed by e-mail. Social media can become an "icebreaker" that may improve the communication between patient and physician, resulting in better patient care [199].

However, this communication via the web is conflicted with a couple of ethical issues since the technologies impact data privacy and security. Gholami-Kordkheili et al. provide a review on the impact of social media on medical professionalism [200]. They identified opportunities and challenges of social media usage in healthcare. Beyond, ethical considerations concerning the relationship between patients and health professionals in the web era were included into the review. These include (1) preserving patient privacy and confidentiality in all environments, (2) avoiding excessive self-disclosure by using adequate privacy settings, and being aware that they are not absolute, and (3) routinely monitoring ones online presence. They claim that appropriate patient/physician boundaries need to be maintained, and in doing so the professional and personal online content should be separated [200].

Further, patient-doctor relationships may suffer from two main situations. On the one hand, patients may have unrestricted access to their doctor's personal information as it is provided on the web. To address this issue, the American Medical Association [37] recommends when using the web for social networking, physicians should use privacy settings to safeguard personal information and content or even better, keep private and professional sectors separately. However, they should realize privacy settings are not absolute and once on the web, content is likely to be there permanently. It is important for physicians and other healthcare professionals to familiarize themselves with the privacy provisions for different social-media applications and adjust the settings to ensure the content is clearly protected.

On the other hand, physicians have access to online patient information that may otherwise not be available in the healthcare setting (e.g. lifestyle information from patients posted in a personal blog). There is a trend to be observed that individuals are recording their personal health data, activity data etc. They are connecting in networks called the "quantified self" to exchange their experiences with health and activities. Using different types of sensors to record weight, blood pressure, sport activity and others, the people's objective is often to become healthier, fitter etc. Such information about a patient received from online sources may be helpful in certain healthcare settings, but physicians need to be sensitive to the source and the way the information was displayed publicly. They should use clinical judgement in determining whether and how to reveal such information during the treatment of patients. Digitally tracking the personal behaviours of patients, such as determining whether they have indeed quit smoking or are maintaining a healthy diet, may threaten the trust needed for a strong patient-physician relationship and have an influence on their treatment of the patient [201].

In summary, physicians must carefully maintain professional relationships and confidentiality in online settings. E-mails and other electronic means of communication may supplement, but not replace face-to-face encounters. Establishing a patient-physician-online relationship, for example to "friend" a patient or ask a patient to "friend" a physician is ethically questionable [201]. The problem results from the fact the professional boundaries of interactions are less clear. Physicians may share personal, but also professional content online. Maintaining professional trust in patient-physician relationships requires physicians to consistently apply ethical principles for preserving the relationship, confidentiality, privacy, and respect for individuals in online settings and mutual communications [202]. Online interactions with patients may pose challenges because of the ambiguity associated with written language without the context of body language or lack of awareness of the potential abuses of social media data [201].

14.3   Implications for Implementing Social Media Applications

In summary, internet-based research and social media usage in healthcare provides new potential risks [4]:

- A patient's privacy might be violated when too much detail about cases are discussed online, especially without the patient's consent,
- Physicians might feel their privacy is violated since more information on them is available than during a patient visit,
- Misunderstandings and misinterpretations through online communication are an issue,
- There is a risk of relying too much on social media and ignoring traditional and more immediate channels of communication.

Privacy issues related to personal and health information are very important in any kind of environment, platform and means of communication (such as electronic health record, e-mail or social media). Several, similar ethical and legal guidelines should be considered in all means of communication and related research. There is no difference between health organisations and researcher when monitoring social media and data exploitation: the same ethical and confidentiality rules must be applied in both cases.

An important point is that, in theory, people know that personal information included in social media platforms, can be shared and accessed by anyone on the web, at least in open platforms. Another important issue is the fact that social media environments can be managed with different profiles and uses, for instance, open groups and closed groups on Facebook have to be managed in a different way in terms of confidentiality and privacy.

Preserving privacy and confidentiality of online users is a main issue as well as providing means for patients or web users to express concerns. For closed groups, the authority from the owner or administrator is necessary before collecting or analysing the data. Using aggregated data by researchers is often acceptable to the community that created it.

Which means and guidelines are available for researcher and clinicians regarding ethical issues of medical social media usage? There are organisations providing guidelines for internet researchers and health professionals. The Association of Internet Researchers (AoIR, http://aoir.org/), provides considerations to support and inform internet researchers about ethical issues [203]. The guidelines comprise a set of questions that should be asked by internet researchers or health organisations when they plan to use social media data for research and monitoring. Questions are addressing issues of potential harms or risks associated with a study, research methods, or storage and representation of collected data.

The American Medical Association (AMA) Code of Medical Ethics provides e-mail guidelines for physicians, which include the necessity to establish a patient-physician relationship in person, using e-mail only for supplemental encounters, and

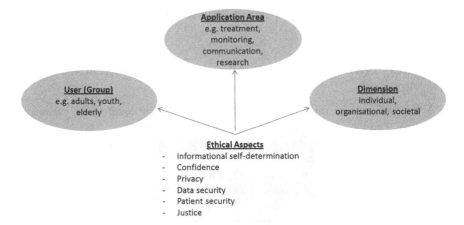

Fig. 14.1 Ethical issues of social media usage in healthcare

informing patients clearly about the inherent limitations of e-mail communication [204]. Also in this guideline, preserving patient privacy and confidentiality in all environments is a main issue.

The European Commission's Information Society Technologies (IST) Programme funded the RESPECT project [205] drew up professional and ethical guidelines for carrying out socio-economic research. The RESPECT guidelines reinforced the methodological challenges associated with online research (identifying dangers of conducting research in this manner) but stopped short of giving specific information tailored to the needs of online communities.

Preserving patient privacy and confidentiality in all environments is a main issue in the context of social media usage in healthcare and research. We tried to raise the important ethical questions related to an appropriate use of social media in healthcare settings. Currently, there are still no official guidelines available that may be applied to address these questions in practice. Given the broad application areas and involved stakeholders, it will be probably impossible to formulate general guidelines for all possible usage scenarios. For each application and research study, researchers and healthcare providers need to carefully weight harm and benefit for the individual patient or groups of patients.

To support such weighting, we suggest a novel model for systematically evaluating technical solutions (see Fig. 14.1). It comprises three aspects. For a concrete social media application in healthcare or medical social media research question, it first need to be clarified which users are involved, which application area is concerned and on which dimension it is operated. Questions include:

- Who is affected by the analysis and application of medical social media data and how should they be affected by it?
- Who is compelled to act on the new knowledge?

- What action is appropriate based on the information learned as a results of the analysis?
- Who is responsible when a predictive analysis is incorrect?

From the answers, ethical issues concerning confidence, privacy, data and patient security or justice may be judged and weighted.

Chapter 15
Integrating Clinical and Social Media Data

Current treatment in healthcare relies upon medical guidelines and medical knowledge that was generalized based on statistical observations of large populations of patients and non-patients. However, the individual state of a patient is much more complex and concerns anatomy, physiology, metabolism, genetics and personal circumstances or life habits [206]. It is characterized by quantitative measurements such as multidimensional images, laboratory results as well as by qualitative information including nutrition habits, physical state, conscience, life style, epigenetic factors etc. Considering the individual state of the patient already in therapy planning is necessary for avoiding complications, predicting possible patient compliance, or for individualizing treatment decisions.

Quantitative measurements as results from examinations are available in the electronic health record, described in clinical narratives or listed in terms of measured values. With an increase of information provision through the Internet, a new source of information reflecting patient's health observations and habits, i.e. qualitative information is increasingly available. Considering both, clinical data and information provided by the patient for example through the use of social media tools could lead to a more close health monitoring and to an individualized care. It could further support in more reliably identifying risk factors, deciding for eligibility for clinical studies, or in monitoring or determining adverse events. However, there are several challenges to be addressed when considering subjective patient judgements possibly derived from medical social media data in treatment planning:

- The quality of the data provided through social media tools is unknown. It can be comprehensive and helpful, but also misleading or wrong.
- Different terminologies and semantics complicate an automatic analysis and interpretation.
- Subjective information needs to be interpreted, weighted and linked to objective clinical parameters.

© Springer International Publishing Switzerland 2015
K. Denecke, *Health Web Science*, Health Information Science,
DOI 10.1007/978-3-319-20582-3_15

- Considering qualitative data provided by the patient in clinical decision making information complicates the aggregation of information and increases the risk of ignoring relevant information.

It becomes clear that when we want to make use of medical social media data to support clinical decision making through consideration of behavioural and social aspects of a patient, we need to find a way to integrate the subjective data with clinical data. In this chapter, we introduce the concept of digital patient modelling as one possibility to integrate the data and to build decision support systems that rely on both, clinical and patient-provided (social media) data. First, the concept of digital patient modelling and model-based decision support is presented followed by the requirements for data integration. Finally, we describe the concept for data integration.

15.1 Digital Patient Modelling and Model-Based Decision Support

The word "model" refers to a *simplified representation of a real-world situation* used to help answering a specific question. Modelling in the domain of healthcare and medicine thus concerns real-world situations in this particular domain. A *digital patient model* can be considered a specific and context-independent representation of a patient or of a specific disease or anatomical structure of a real patient, respectively. It consists of data elements that are semantically linked or grouped and thus provides an integrated view on the patient data reflecting his health status.

Several data items are generated during a healthcare treatment process. Normally, the data available comprises texts, images or recorded speech in form of diagnostic reports, CT-scans, biosignals, 2D-, 3D-, or 4D-models as well as simulation models. Since the data is recorded by different medical devices, there are many specialized information systems and isolated data items. The physician needs to consult the various systems in order to get a complete view on the patient's state. Given this distributed and heterogeneous nature of data, there is a high risk of missing or misjudging important information items. A digital patient model addresses this problem by integrating the relevant information related to a disease or anatomical structure including morphological, functional, static or dynamic data. Information from various types (image data, structured data etc.) is integrated in a reasonable manner in a patient-specific model. It can further describe relations between clinical parameters and sociological factors related to a specific clinical pathology. Patient models occur in various facets [207]:

1. Geometric patient models (e.g., 3D-images/3D patient model of a specific organ such as 3D panendoscopy or patient-specific modelling of the heart),
2. Dynamic or functional patient models (e.g. blood flow),

3. Patient models for diagnosis (e.g. presentation characteristics of esophagus cancer [208], causal probabilistic model for diagnosis of bacterial urinary tract infection [209]),
4. Predictive patient models for disease progress or therapy planning.

A digital patient model can be exploited in multiple ways. Integrated in a decision support system it can support in therapy planning with individual quantitative optimization of clinical output or in predicting disease propagation. Treatment options can be simulated to support decision making.

More specifically, a model-based decision support system exploits digital patient models and bases upon two assumptions [210]:

1. Medical knowledge can be modelled including diagnosis, treatment, and decision making processes, i.e. it can be formally described which parameters characterize a specific diagnosis or which steps are performed within a decision-making process. We refer to this medical knowledge as domain theory or knowledge layer.
2. The observations made during physical or other clinical assessment of a patient can be described and instantiates the formal patient model. We refer to this by the term situation description comprising the information and data layer. The information model layer concerns the representation and storage of clinical data. For achieving interoperability among information systems as well as a high level of standardization of clinical data exchange the underlying information model needs to be the same. The data layer of a model-based decision support systems comprises integrated data items from the same or from different data types. On the data layer, a digital patient model integrates the relevant data items related to a disease or anatomical structure including morphological, functional, static or dynamic data.

At the knowledge layer, a digital patient model comprises data structures and methods to describe an organ or disease by characteristic information items and mathematical relations among them. An integration of the knowledge layer with the information and patient-specific data layer enables to build patient-specific models to be considered in decision making and planning (Fig. 15.1).

Consider the following example: A decision support system for treatment decisions of laryngeal carcinoma bases upon a structural model (i.e. the knowledge layer) describing parameters to be considered in decision making (e.g. information entities such as age or extracapsular spread of lymph node metastasis). For each information entity (attribute) a value describing the normal state is assigned and also probabilities to what extent the entity contributes to the decision process. During situation assessment, the attributes of the model are instantiated with the measured data from the information and data layers. A decision support system could use that information together with the structural model to predict the outcome for various treatment options. In the following, we are collecting requirements for data integration using digital patient models.

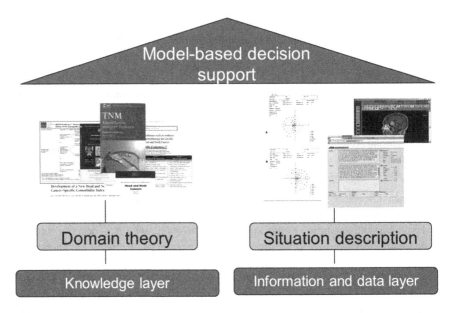

Fig. 15.1 A model-based decision support system bases upon a data layer, an information layer and a knowledge layer

15.2 Requirements for Data Integration

Integration of clinical data with medical social media data has several requirements that can be grouped into (1) functional requirements, (2) semantic requirements and (3) technical requirements (see Table 15.1).

Considering a user's perspective, there are several functional requirements. Clearly, all relevant data need to be available and accessible. Since the patient model is supposed to integrate different data item generated by multiple authors and collected from clinical and social media sources, metainformation on the data needs to be available, e.g., on data source, by whom some data was provided, the date of provision, information on the methods with which some data was measured etc. Since many data items are available, in particular when a patient is monitored and treated for a longer time period, methods for automatically analysing data are required to facilitate human analysis and interpretation. This also includes methods for reasoning and inference to draw automatically conclusions and generate alerts for a physician for example when a patient's health status changed significantly.

Semantic requirements include standardized, normalized storage of data and relations between data items. Data need to be represented in a way that allows search and analysis, i.e. unstructured texts need to be structured and multimedia data need to be semantically annotated to enable retrieval and data linking. As we have seen, one option is to map unstructured text to concepts of a biomedical ontology. Radiological images or other non-textual data items can be tagged with

Table 15.1 Requirements for data integration

Functional requirements	Semantic requirements	Technical requirements
• Availability of metainformation • Facilities for automatic analysis and interpretation • Methods for reasoning and inference • Retrieval facilities	• Integrated information with related information items • Dynamic adaptation over time • Semantic annotation with ontologies • Distinction between historical and current data • Structured representation of data	• Data storage • Multimodal retrieval methods for integrated data of different types • Natural language processing for automatically analysing clinical and social media data

biomedical concepts. In particular, specific patho-physiological structures could be explicitly annotated. Additionally, qualitative information has to be represented in a standardized, interpretable manner and also linked to quantitative data. Historical data need to be separated from current data since its interpretation within a current treatment may differ. Beyond, metadata on data items is necessary, for example information on the reliability of the respective data item (e.g. by indicating the source of information: social media versus electronic health record) or on the phase in which a data item was acquired (before, between or after a surgery). Semantic relations are necessary to link data items, e.g. images to images, text to images, values to text. This requires identification of relations among information items. Such relations can be manifested in a time span (e.g. data that was produced during the same time period is likely to be related), a medical condition, a treatment or others.

Technical requirements of data integration comprise a data representation that is easy to query and store. Natural language processing methods are necessary to analyse and process unstructured, free textual data, for searching, comparing, summarizing to enable research, improve standards of care and evaluate outcomes. Machine learning methods allow for automatic analysis, classification and clustering. We believe that creating a digital patient model offers the opportunity to consider these requirements and to integrate information from medical social media and electronic health records.

15.3 Data Integration Using Digital Patient Modelling

A frequently used method for knowledge modelling within clinical decision support systems are Bayesian networks which are probabilistic graphical models (e.g. Oniko et al. [211], Leibovici et al. [209]). Random variables represent in these graphs information entities such as medical examinations, medical imaging, patient behaviour and patient characteristics (e.g. age, gender, tobacco and alcohol consumption), while directed edges represent the dependencies between information entities. Conditional probabilities need to be set for each information entity based on the graphical model structure. They define the correlation between an information and its direct causes. Bayesian networks allow for example to model dependencies among relevant information entities with respect to treatment decisions [212].

Within a clinical decision support system, such probabilistic models allow to

- Model dependencies among relevant information entities with respect to treatment decisions [212],
- Simulate processes,
- Provide objective judgements of different treatment options, or
- Point to missing information entities.

15.3.1   Generating Probabilistic Graphical Models

So far, clinical simulation and planning using Bayesian networks has been performed on generic models created using heuristics, which clearly lack information on the individual patient, his or her personal state and characteristic physiology. General models are well suited for education or training purposes. To generate a general Bayesian network for a disease, a graphical model needs to be created and probabilities must be set. For the graphical model, relevant information entities and their dependencies have to be collected. This can be realised by applying natural language processing algorithms to a set of relevant clinical guidelines, biomedical literature and other relevant documents to extract information entities and their relations. Additionally, machine learning can be applied to structured patient case data to learn variables and identify relations between them. These sources already provide the probabilities that are necessary for the model generation as well [213]. Antal et al. [214] suggest for example an approach to learn Bayesian networks for the classification of ovarian tumours from literature and data. They extract relevant information from documents using text mining and apply statistical methods to derive pair wise dependency measures. Once the graphical model is completed, conditional probabilities need to be assigned, either manually or learnt from data.

15.3.2   From a General Model to Patient-Specific Models

For prognosis and prediction of individual outcomes, patient-specific parameters, i.e. a patient-specific Bayesian network is necessary. The general model thus needs to be instantiated with patient-specific parameters which can be clinical

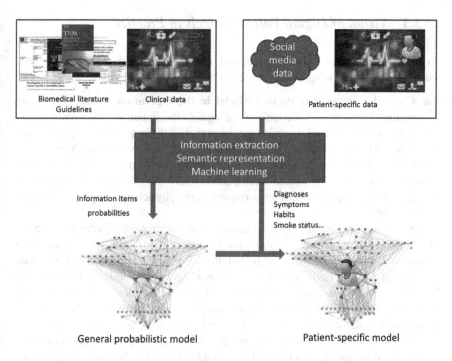

Fig. 15.2 To identify information entities and their dependencies required for creating a general probabilistic graphical model, information extraction and machine learning methods can be applied to clinical data, guidelines and biomedical literature. A patient-specific model is created by instantiating a general probabilistic model with data extracted from the electronic health records and medical social media data

parameters, but also qualitative information derived from patient-specific social media data or other healthcare data provided by the patient. Using analysis methods as presented in this book, relevant information can be extracted from patient-specific medical social media data and from the electronic health record (Fig. 15.2).

In this way, a digital patient model could provide a mean to integrate social media and clinical data by considering or representing the relevant information extracted from social media reflecting the patient health status in corresponding nodes. In addition to clinical data, social media could provide information on social factors, behaviour, environmental factors which can be included into a digital patient model and thus included into decision making. This can be achieved by extending the underlying general model by nodes and dependencies representing relevant social, behaviour and environmental factors. The conditional probabilities need to be assigned accordingly to reflect the different weights of the information types.

15.3.3 Vision of Digital Patient Models in Practice

To demonstrate use cases for digital patient models that include social media data, we consider the following futuristic scenarios.

Use Case: An Integrated Patient Model in the Operation Room A surgeon is operating a tumour and recognizes that against the initial planning and appearances in the radiological images, the tumour size is larger than expected and lymph nodes are affected. In order to decide about the following procedure, several questions need to be answered and require information from the electronic health record or patient-specific patient model, respectively. This information is provided by the decision support system upon request of the physician through direct verbal communication.

First, he is dictating the updated tumour size information: "Tumour size 5cm, two lymph nodes are affected, suspicion of metastasis". The system updates the patient model and recalculates the probabilities for the therapeutic decision. Given the adapted conditions, the algorithms provide a higher probability for radiotherapy. Therefore, the system recommends this intervention. The physician is asking for reasons for this decision and the system explains: "Good general condition, young men, family status: married, job as health care worker, non-smoking". The physician would like to verify these reasons and gets presented snippets from documents where the data has been extracted with highlighting of the relevant passages. Beyond, it is checking in the background for similar patient cases that are stored as digital patient model. It provides the information that from the found similar cases, 87 % of the patients with similar characteristics were successfully treated by applying radiotherapy. Storing these justifications, the surgeon asks the system to update the treatment: he will stop the operation and revise the therapy.

In this scenario, the model-based decision support system has to provide relevant information, update the patient-specific model depending on the situation and make adapted treatment suggestions considering the new situations. The following scenario exploits the patient model as basis for information retrieval and information provision.

Use Case: Information Retrieval and Provision Since a digital patient model reflects the health status of a patient with respect to an organ or medical condition at some point of time, it can be assumed that it can form the basis for determining the information need of a physician or patient. The underlying hypothesis is that physician or patient are searching for information related to the disease, in particular for information on decision-relevant information items. A retrieval system based on a patient-specific model could determine decision-relevant parameters by identifying the nodes in the Bayesian network that have the largest impact on the therapy options or on other nodes. For the resulting information items, biomedical literature, patient information or other information could be automatically retrieved. Even one step further, digital patient models for patients that have been treated by a physician could characterize his expertise. When searching for an expert, the result set could be determined by finding similar patient models. Physicians with similar patient models for treated patients could be suggested as relevant for linking in a social network. Altogether, this could result in a medical, evidence-based and social semantic desktop for different user groups (patients and physicians/health carers).

These scenarios show the potentials of digital patient modelling and integration of medical social media with clinical practice. There is still a lot to do to realise these or similar scenarios. This book intended to provide a starting point for their realisation. However, a very interesting and challenging research journey still lies ahead of us and will lead us into the future of Health Web Science.

Chapter 16
Concluding Remarks

At the beginning of the book, we raised several theoretical and practical questions associated with Health Web Science as considered in this book. We will briefly summarise the results.

Theoretical Questions About the Nature of Medical Social Media Data: Medical social media data is characterised by experiential information on diseases, treatments and drug consumption. Besides, lifestyle information is provided. Language differs from clinical documents with respect to the frequently used word classes including a frequent use of verbs and pronouns, non-medical named entities and a large variety in adjectives.

Theoretical Questions About Analysing Social Media Data: Existing clinical information extraction tools are suited for analysing medical social media texts when sentences are not too complex and medical terms are exploited. Tools would need to be extended by analysis methods for verbs, personal pronouns, adjectives and coordinating structures. Open information extraction methods have a potential for addressing the limitation of current information extraction tools with respect to the analysis of verbs and associated relations. Methods need to be developed suited for analysing the medical sentiment in medical social media data and clinical data. Many applications are possible.

Practical Questions of Implementing Social Media in Healthcare: Most crucial ethical and legal aspects regarding the use of medical social media data are related to privacy, authenticity and the impact on the patient-doctor relationship. Ethical aspects of Internet-based research studies and social media applications may be appropriately judged and weighted considering user group, application area and dimension.

Finally, we conclude with some critical remarks on the analyses in this book. It is clear that an assessment as we described it in this book can only consider a subset of medical social media data. The data set underlying our study mainly comprised blogs mainly written by health professionals. The content is thus more informa-

© Springer International Publishing Switzerland 2015
K. Denecke, *Health Web Science*, Health Information Science,
DOI 10.1007/978-3-319-20582-3_16

tional; information on medical treatments are described. Content and language could be different when only patient-written blogs are considered. A generalization of the results to patient-written texts is difficult. It might be that patient-written blogs present also clinical data or at least personal judgements and observations of the health status. It would be interesting to run a similar analysis on different medical social media types contributed by different author groups. An extended linguistic analysis of medical blogs could concentrate on verb usage, which was studied for medical corpora already [215]. Wang et al. studied operative notes and their content and language by analysing and categorising verbs [216]. An alternative approach to study differences between language and content in clinical notes of different types and specialities was suggested by Patterson and Hurdle [217]. They proposed a document clustering approach to study in more detail characteristics of clinical sublanguages. To determine patterns of semantic types, we applied open information extraction, which was so far not considered for sublanguage analysis. We decided to use that approach to be able to extract the relation type. This goes beyond co-occurrence analysis of semantic types and is interesting, since verb meanings would get lost during the mapping process to UMLS. A limitation of this approach is that only relations with two arguments are extracted by the chosen implementation. Corpus analysis methods [218] would be an additional option for analysing medical social media data. We chose sublanguage analysis to be able to compare with results from sublanguage analysis from clinical texts.

Glossary

Blog A blog or weblog is a discussion or informational site published on the web and consisting of discrete entries ("posts") typically displayed in reverse chronological order.

Coreference resolution Coreference resolution is the task of finding all expressions that refer to the same entity in a text.

Digital patient model A digital patient model can be considered a specific and context-independent representation of a patient or of a specific disease or anatomical structure of a real patient, respectively. It consists of data elements that are semantically linked or grouped and thus provides an integrated view on the patient data.

Diversity Diversity is introduced as measure for dissimilarity. Result diversification is realised by finding the best trade off between diversity and similarity [172]. It targets finding the right balance between having more relevant results of the "correct" intent and having more diverse results in the top positions [173, 174].

Ethics Ethics concerns two basic practical problems of human life: (1) What is worth seeking—that is, what goals of life are good? and (2) What individuals are responsible for—that is, what duties should they recognize and attempt to fulfil [192].

© Springer International Publishing Switzerland 2015
K. Denecke, *Health Web Science*, Health Information Science,
DOI 10.1007/978-3-319-20582-3

Event	An event is a significant change in the state of a situation, environment or person. Whether a change is significant depends on the user.
False positive	A false positive is defined as an alert that is raised in the absence of a real world event.
Forum	A forum or internet forum is a public discussion place in the web.
Health Web Science	Health Web Science is the medico-socio-technical science that investigates how the web evolves with respect to health issues, how health related data provided through the web can be processed and how tools that make use of web technology can be used in healthcare.
Information extraction	Information extraction is the identification, and consequent or concurrent classification and structuring into semantic classes, of specific information found in unstructured data sources, such as natural language text, making the information more suitable for information processing tasks.
Indicator	An indicator is a hint to an event. For example the number of documents mentioning some specific term is an indicator.
Medical ethics	Medical ethics concentrates on ethical issues regarding the relationship between patients and doctors.
Medical social media	Medical social media data is a subset of the social media data space, in which the interests of the participants are specifically devoted to medicine and health issues.
Metadata	Metadata is data about data. Structural metadata describes the design and specification of data structures. Descriptive metadata is about individual instances of application data or the data content.
Monitoring	Monitoring is the active or passive routine collection of information on an object or process with the purpose of detecting changes over time.

Natural language processing (NLP)	Natural language processing encompasses a range of computational techniques for analysing and representing natural language texts. They target at making unstructured data available for a range of tasks or applications.
Open information extraction	Open information extraction (open IE, [61, 102]) is the task of extracting assertions from massive corpora without requiring a pre-specified vocabulary. It identifies phrases that denote relations in sentences. The extraction avoids the problem of being restricted to a pre-specified vocabulary.
Ontology	An ontology is a set of concepts relevant to a particular area of interest.
Part of speech (POS)	A POS is the linguistic category of a word.
Part of speech tagger	A POS tagger is a tool that assigns a word class to a word.
Parsing	Parsing is the process of breaking down a sentence into its constituents parts. A full parser connects all words and phrases together into a sentence while a shallow parser combines words into noun phrases, verb phrases and prepositional phrases, but resists on linking the phrases together.
Podcast	A podcast is a digital medium to which a person can subscribe to and content can be downloaded through web syndication or streamed on-line to a computer or mobile device. The content consists of an episodic series of audio, video, digital radio, PDF, or ePub files.
Public health ethics	Public health ethics deals with the specific moral questions regarding public actions for disease prevention, life elongation, or psychological and physical well-being.
Review portal	A review portal in the web allows to rate persons, services or objects according to certain criteria or in free-textual comments.

Really Simple Syndication	RSS is a family of web feed formats used to publish frequently updated works.
Sentiment analysis	Sentiment analysis or opinion mining refers to methods that identify, extract and analyse subjective information in texts. Typical tasks is the classification of texts as positive or negative.
Signal	A signal is created when an event of relevance is detected, for example when a number of daily counts exceeds some threshold.
Situational awareness	Situational awareness is the ability to identify, process, and comprehend the critical elements of information about what is happening to the team with regards to the mission.
Social media	Social media is defined as "a group of Internet-based applications that build on the ideological and technological foundations of Web 2.0, and that allow the creation and exchange of user-generated content" [219].
Social text stream	Social text streams are defined as collection of informal text communication distributed over the web. Each piece of text is associated with social attributes such as author.
Social sensor	A social sensor is any source of information that can be identified in Web 2.0 tools. In such sources, situations and facts about users are expressed either by the user himself, by others or just through his interaction with these tools. Examples of social sensors include Twitter posts, Facebook status updates or pictures posted on Flickr.
Stream	To a set of continuously arriving events we refer as a stream.
Sublanguage	Sublanguage is the language of a restricted domain, for example the medical domain, and in this way a subset of a natural language characterized by the fact that only a subset of the vocabulary and certain grammatical rules are used.

Sublanguage analysis   Sublanguage analysis is a technique for discovering units of information and their relationships in narrative text.

Surveillance   Surveillance is the systematic, continuous monitoring of objects, persons or situations.

Surveillance system   Surveillance systems monitor, track and assess the movements of individuals, their property and other assets.

Textanalytic-enabled system   A textanalytic-enabled system is an application that analyses textual social media data for their exploitation in healthcare.

Time series   A time series is a sequence of observations made over time.

Transfer learning   Transfer learning or inductive learning is a research problem in machine learning that focuses on storing knowledge gained while solving one problem and applying it to a different but related problem.

Unified Medical Language System   The UMLS integrates and distributes key biomedical terminology, classification and coding standards, and provides associated resources. It is curated by the National Library of Medicine.

User-generated content   User-generated content is any form of web content such as blogs, wikis, discussion forums, posts, chats, tweets, podcasting, that was created by users of an online system or service, often made available via social media websites.

Vlog   A video blog is a form of blog where content is provided as video.

Web mining   Web mining targets at finding patterns in web data. It comprises the tasks web usage mining, web content mining and web structure mining.

Web Science   "Web Science must be inherently interdisciplinary; its
                               goal is both, to understand the growth of the web and to
                               create approaches that allow new powerful and more
                               beneficial patterns to occur" [2].

Wiki   A wiki is a type of content management system. Being
                               typically a web application, it allows collaborative
                               modification, extension, or deletion of its content and
                               structure. In a typical wiki, text is written using a
                               simplified markup language or a rich-text editor.

References

1. Ben Shneiderman. Web science: a provocative invitation to computer science. *Commun. ACM*, 50(6):25–27, June 2007.
2. Tim Berners-Lee, Wendy Hall, James Hendler, Nigel Shadbolt, and Daniel J. Weitzner. Creating a science of the web. *Science*, 313:769–71, 2006.
3. Elizabeth H. Brooks, Grant P. Cumming, and Joanne S. Luciano. Health web science: application of web science to the area of health education and health care. In *Proceedings of the second international workshop on Web science and information exchange in the medical web*, MedEx '11, pages 11–14, New York, NY, USA, 2011. ACM.
4. P. Eckler, G. Worsowicz, and J.W. Rayburn. Social media and health care: an overview. *PM R.*, 2(11):1046–50, 2010.
5. P. Wicks, M. Massagli, J. Frost, and et al. Sharing health data for better outcomes on patientslikeme. *J Med Internet Res*, 12(2), 2010.
6. T. Lagu, E.J. Kaufman, D.A. Asch, and K. Armstrong. Content of weblogs written by health professionals. *J Gen Intern Med.*, 23(10):164–76, 2008.
7. G. Eysenbach. Medicine 2.0: social networking, collaboration, participation, apomediation, and openness. *J Med Internet Res.*, 10(3), 2008.
8. Ves Dimov. Casesblog - medical and health blog. health news updated daily by internist and allergist at cleveland clinic. http://casesblog.blogspot.de/, last accessed: 14.03.2015.
9. Kevin Pho. Kevinmd. http://www.kevinmd.com/blog/, last accessed: 14.03.2015.
10. Mayo Clinic. Mayo clinic youtube channel. http://www.youtube.com/user/mayoclinic, last accessed: 14.03.2015.
11. Mayo Clinic. Health care social media list. http://network.socialmedia.mayoclinic.org/hcsml-grid/, last accessed: 14.03.2015.
12. S. Fox. Health topics. pew research center's internet and american life project. http://www.pewinternet.org/~/media//Files/Reports/2011/PIP_Health_Topics.pdf, 2011. last accessed: 20.03.2013.
13. K. Denecke and A. Stewart. Learning from medical social media data: current state and future challenges. In *In: White B, King I, Tsang P, editors. Social Media Tools and Platforms in Learning Environments*, pages 353–372, 2011.
14. A.Y. Lau, K.A. Siek, L. Fernandez-Luque, and et al. The role of social media for patients and consumer health. *Yearb Med Inform.*, 6:131–8, 2011.
15. Stephanie Medlock, Saeid Eslami, Marjan Askari, Danielle Sent, Sophia E. de Rooij, and Ameen Abu-Hanna. The consequences of seniors seeking health information using the internet and other sources. *Studies in Health Technology and Informatics*, 192:457–60, 2013.

© Springer International Publishing Switzerland 2015
K. Denecke, *Health Web Science*, Health Information Science,
DOI 10.1007/978-3-319-20582-3

16. E. Velasco, T. Agheneza, K. Denecke, G. Kirchner, and T. Eckmanns. Social media and internet-based data in global systems for public health surveillance: A systematic review. *Milbank Quarterly*, 92(1):7–33, 2014.

17. L. Aase, D. Goldman, M. Gould, J. Noseworthy, and F. Timimi. *Bringing the Social-media Revolution to Health Care*. Mayo Clinic Center for Social-media, 2012.

18. J. Stinson, L. Jibb, P. Nathan, and et al. Development and testing of a multidimensional iphone pain assessment application for adolescents with cancer. iPROCEEDINGS Medicine 2.0 Boston, Sept 15–16 2012. http://www.medicine20congres.com, http://www.medicine20congress.com/ocs/index.php/med/med2012/paper/view/910.

19. S. Khairat and C. Garcia. Introducing a wireless mobile technology to improve diabetes care outcomes among specific minority groups. iPROCEEDINGS Medicine 2.0 Boston, Sept 15–16 2012. http://www.medicine20congres.com, http://www.medicine20congress.com/ocs/index.php/med/med2012/paper/view/900.

20. W.H. Ho, P. Weinstein, D. De Sousa, and et al. A mobile clinical collaboration system for inter-professional team based care in an outpatient setting. iPROCEEDINGS Medicine 2.0 Boston, Sept 15–16 2012. http://www.medicine20congres.com, http://www.medicine20congress.com/ocs/index.php/med/med2012/paper/view/1243.

21. L.L. Struik, J.L. Bottorff, Jung, and C. M. Budgen. Facebook me: The use of social networking sites for gender-sensitive tobacco control messaging. iPROCEEDINGS Medicine 2.0 Boston, Sept 15–16 2012. http://www.medicine20congres.com, http://www.medicine20congress.com/ocs/index.php/med/med2012/paper/view/785.

22. Simon McCallum. Gamification and serious games for personalized health. In *B. Blobel (ed.) pHealth 2012*, pages 85–90. IOS Press, 2012.

23. G. Llinas, D. Rodriguez-Inesta, J.J. Mira, S. Lorenzo, and C. Aibar. A comparison of websites from spanish, american and british hospitals. *Methods Inf Med*, 47 (2):124–130, 2008.

24. Pew Internet Project. Health fact sheet. http://www.pewinternet.org/fact-sheets/health-fact-sheet/, last accessed: 14.03.2015.

25. T. Greenhalgh. Patient and public involvement in chronic illness: beyond the expert patient. *BMJ*, 338, 2009.

26. S.L. Ayers and J.J. Kronenfeld. Chronic illness and health-seeking information on the internet. *Health*, 11 (3):327–347, 2007.

27. J. Moreland, T.L. French, and G.P. Cumming. To what extent are people using the internet to obtain health information in the uk: How online health seeking behaviour influences offline behaviour among patients. In *Proceedings of Medicine 2.0: Social Media and Web 2.0 (Medicine 2.0). Harvard Medical School, Boston, USA*, 2012.

28. DailyStrength. Dailystrength depression support group. http://www.dailystrength.org/c/Depression/support-group, last accessed: 14.03.2015.

29. Docsboard. Docsboard: Dicussion board for doctors. http://www.docsboard.com, last accessed: 14.03.2015.

30. HON. Health on the net foundation. http://www.hon.ch, last accessed: 14.03.2015.

31. P.M. Archambault, T.H. Van De Belt, F.J. Grajales Iii, and et al. Wikis and collaborative writing applications in health care: Preliminary results of a scoping review. iPROCEEDINGS Medicine 2.0 Boston, Sept 15–16 2012. http://www.medicine20congres.com, http://www.medicine20congress.com/ocs/index.php/med/med2012/paper/view/994.

32. Patient Opinion. Patient opinion. https://www.patientopinion.org.uk, last accessed: 14.03.2015.

33. B.H. Walter. Telling tales: Treatment stories on an eating disorder support websites. iPROCEEDINGS Medicine 2.0 Boston, Sept 15–16 2012. http://www.medicine20congres.com, http://www.medicine20congress.com/ocs/index.php/med/med2012/paper/view/924.

34. AskaPatient. Ask a patient. http://www.askapatient.com/, last accessed: 14.03.2015.

35. C.A. Brownstein, J.S. Brownstein, D.S. Williams, and et al. The power of social networking in medicine. *Nature Biotechnology*, 27:888–890, 2009.

36. K. Denecke, M. Krieck, L. Otrusina, and et al. How to exploit twitter for public health monitoring? *Methods of Information in Medicine*, 52(4):326–39, 2013.

37. Diane J. Standiford. A stellarlife. http://dj-astellarlife.blogspot.de, last accessed: 14.03.2015.
38. Randy Pausch. Randy pausch's update page. http://www.cs.cmu.edu/~pausch/news/index. html, last accessed: 14.03.2015.
39. Amy Tenderich. Diabetesmine. http://www.diabetesmine.com/, last accessed: 14.03.2015.
40. WebMD. Webmd website. http://www.webmd.com, last accessed: 14.03.2015.
41. EveryDayHealth. Every day health media. http://www.everydayhealth.com, last accessed: 14.03.2015.
42. WebMD. Medicinenet. http://www.medicinenet.com, last accessed: 14.03.2015.
43. DrugRatingz. Drugratingz. http://www.drugratingz.com/, last accessed: 14.03.2015.
44. Slashdot. Slashdot. http://slashdot.org, last accessed: 14.03.2015.
45. Medical Coding Consultants. Ritecode. http://www.ritecode.com/free_opreports/opreport_ free_index.htm, last accessed: 10.2.2013.
46. NHS. Nhs choices. http://nhs.uk, last accessed: 14.03.2015.
47. Mayo Clinic. Mayo clinic. http://www.mayoclinic.com, last accessed: 14.03.2015.
48. DiabetesDaily. Diabetes daily. http://www.diabetesdaily.com/forum/, last accessed: 14.03.2015.
49. K. Denecke and W. Nejdl. How valuable is medical social media data? content analysis of the medical web. *Journal of Information Science*, 179:1870–1880, 2009.
50. Myca Health. Hellohealth. https://hellohealth.com/solutions/patient-portal/, last accessed: 14.03.2015.
51. PatientsLikeMe. Patientslikeme. http://www.patientslikeme.com/, last accessed: 14.03.2015.
52. RateMD. Ratemd. http://www.ratemds.com/, last accessed: 14.03.2015.
53. Z. Harris. *A theory of language and information: a mathematical approach*. Clarendon Press, Oxford, 1991.
54. Carol Friedman, Pauline Kra, and Andrey Rzhetsky A. Two biomedical sublanguages: a description based on the theories of zellig harris. *Journal of Biomedical Informatics*, 35:222–235, 2002.
55. D. A. Campbell and S. B. Johnson. Comparing syntactic complexity in medical and non-medical corpora. *Proc AMIA Symp*, pages 90–94, 2001.
56. Naomi Sager and Ngo Thanh Nhan. The computability of strings, transformations, and sublanguage. In Bruce E. Nevin and Stephen M. Johnson, editors, *The legacy of Zellig Harris: Language and information into the 21st century*, pages 79–120. John Benjamins, 2002.
57. Ivor Kovic, Ileana Lulic, and Gordana Brumini. Examining the Medical Blogosphere: An Online Survey of Medical Bloggers. *Journal of Medical Internet Research*, 10(3), 2008.
58. S.M. Meystre, G.K. Savova, K.C. Kipper-Schuler, and J.F: Hurdle. Extracting information from textual documents in the electronic health record: a review of recent research. *Yearbook Med Informat*, pages 128–44, 2008.
59. Marcus Mitchell. Penn tree pos tagger. http://www.cis.upenn.edu/~treebank/, last accessed: 14.03.2015.
60. Theresa Wilson, Janyce Wiebe, and Paul Hoffmann. Recognizing contextual polarity in phrase-level sentiment analysis. In *Proceedings of the Conference on Human Language Technology and Empirical Methods in Natural Language Processing*, HLT '05, pages 347–354, Stroudsburg, PA, USA, 2005. Association for Computational Linguistics.
61. Anthony Fader, Stephen Soderland, and Oren Etzioni. Identifying relations for open information extraction. In *Proceedings of the Conference on Empirical Methods in Natural Language Processing*, EMNLP '11, pages 1535–1545, Stroudsburg, PA, USA, 2011. Association for Computational Linguistics.
62. X. Zhou, X. Zhang, and X. Hu. Dragon toolkit: Incorporating auto-learned semantic knowledge into large-scale text retrieval and mining. In *Proceedings of the 19th IEEE International Conference on Tools with Artificial Intelligence (ICTAI), October 29–31, 2007, Patras, Greece*, 2007.
63. Kerstin Denecke and Yihan Deng. Sentiment analysis in medical settings - new opportunities and challenges. *Artificial Intelligence in Medicine*, 2015.
64. OpenCalais. Opencalais website. http://www.opencalais.com, last accessed: 14.03.2015.

65. S. Bird, E Klein, and E. Loper. *Natural Language Processing with Python*. O'Reilly Media Inc., http://www.nltk.org/book, 2009.
66. Montylingua. Montylingua: A free, commonsense-enriched natural language understander for english. http://web.media.mit.edu/~hugo/montylingua/, last accessed: 14.03.2015.
67. LingPipe. Alias-i: Lingpipe. http://alias-i.com/lingpipe/, last accessed: 14.03.2015.
68. T. Obrebski and M. Stolarski. Uam text tools - a flexible nlp architecture. In *Proceedings of LREC 2006, Genova*, 2006.
69. C. Grover and et al. A framework for text mining services. In *Proceedings of the Third UK e-Science Programme All Hands Meeting (AHM 2004)*, page 67, 2004.
70. A. Ferrucci and A. Lally. Uima: an architectural approach to unstructured information processing in the corporate research environment. *Natural Language Engineering*, 10:327–48, 2006.
71. Guergana K. Savova, James J. Masanz, Philip V. Ogren, Jiaping Zheng, Sunghwan Sohn, Karin C. Kipper-Schuler, and Christopher G. Chute. Mayo clinical text analysis and knowledge extraction system (ctakes): architecture, component evaluation and applications. *J Am Med Inform Assoc*, 17:507–513, 2010.
72. H. Cunningham. Gate, a general architecture for text engineering. *Computers and the Humanities*, 36:223–254, 2002.
73. Siddhartha Jonnalagadda, Trevor Cohen, Stephen Wu, and Graciela Gonzalez. Enhancing clinical concept extraction with distributional semantics. *Journal of Biomedical Informatics*, 45(1):129–140, 2012.
74. W.R. Hersh. *Information Retrieval: A Health and Biomedical Perspective*. Springer-Verlag, 2003.
75. S.M. Weiss, N. Indurkhya, T. Zhang, and F.J. Damerau. *Text Mining: Predictive Methods for Analysing Unstructured Information*. Springer-Verlag, 2004.
76. Jim Cowie and Wendy Lehnert. Information extraction. *Commun. ACM*, 39(1):80–91, January 1996.
77. R. Grisham. Chapter 30: Information extraction. In *Mitkov R: The Oxford Handbook of Computational Linguistics*. Oxford University Press, 2002.
78. Ralph Grishman. Information extraction and speech recognition. In *Proceedings of the Broadcast News Transcription and Understanding Workshop, Lansdowne, VA*, 1998.
79. Aaron Cohen and William Hersh. A survey of current work in biomedical text mining. *Brief Bioinform*, 6(1):57–71, January 2005.
80. National Library of Medicine. Unified medical language system. http://www.nlm.nih.gov/research/umls/, last accessed: 14.03.2015.
81. Alexa T. McCray. An upper-level ontology for the biomedical domain. *Comp Funct Genom*, 4:80–84, 2003.
82. A. Burgun A.T. McCray and O. Bodenreider. Aggregating umls semantic types for reducing conceptual complexity. In *Stud Health Technol Inform.*, pages 216–220, 2001.
83. National Library of Medicine. Medical subject headings. http://www.nlm.nih.gov/pubs/factsheets/mesh.html, last accessed: 14.03.2015.
84. IHTSDO Organisation. International health terminology standards development organisation. http://www.ihtsdo.org/snomed-ct/snomed-ct0/, last accessed: 14.03.2015.
85. Stanford NLP. Stanford named entity recognizer. http://nlp.stanford.edu/software/CRF-NER.shtml, last accessed: 14.03.2015.
86. J. Friedlin and C.J. McDonald. A natural language processing system to extract and code concepts relating to congestive heart failure from chest radiology reports. *AMIA Annu Symp Proc.*, pages 269–73, 2006.
87. D.T. Heinze B.W. Mamlin and C.J. McDonald. Automated extraction and normalization of findings from cancer-related free-text radiology reports. *AMIA Annu Symp Proc.*, pages 420–4, 2003.
88. C. Friedman, P.O. Alderson, J.H. Austin, J.J. Cimino, and S.B. Johnson. A general natural-language text processor for clinical radiology. *J Am Med Inform Assoc.*, 1(2):161–174, 1994.

89. Alan R. Aronson. Effective mapping of biomedical text to the umls metathesaurus: The metamap program. In *Proceedings of the AMIA 2001*, 2001.

90. Carol Friedman, Thomas C. Rindflesch, and Milton Corn. Natural language processing: State of the art and prospects for significant progress, a workshop sponsored by the national library of medicine. *Journal of Biomedical Informatics*, 46(5):765–773, 2013.

91. G. Savova, S. Bethard, W. Styler, J. Martin, M. Palmer, J. Masanz, and W. Ward. Towards temporal relation discovery from the clinical narrative. In *AMIA Annual Symposium Proceedings*, volume 2009, page 568. American Medical Informatics Association, American Medical Informatics Association, 2009.

92. Jörn Kottman. Apache opennlp. https://opennlp.apache.org/, last accessed: 14.03.2015.

93. Karin Kipper-Schuler, Vinod Kaggal, James Masanz, Philip Ogren, and Guergana Savova. System evaluation on a named entity corpus from clinical notes. In *Language Resources and Evaluation Conference, LREC 2008*, pages 3001–7, 2008.

94. Gunther Schadow and Clement J. McDonald. Extracting structured information from free text pathology reports. *AMIA Annu Symp Proc.*, pages 584–588, 2003.

95. W.W. Chapman, M. Fiszman, J.N. Dowling, B.E. Chapman, and T.C. Rindflesch. Identifying respiratory findings in emergency department reports for biosurveillance using metamap. In *Stud Health Technol Inform.*, pages 487–91, 2004.

96. M.E. von Maltzahn S.A. Stewart and S.S. Raza Abidi. Comparing metamap to mgrep as a tool for mapping free text to formal medical lexions. In *Proceedings of the 1st International Workshop on Knowledge Extraction and Consolidation from Social-media in conjunction with the 11th International Semantic Web Conference (ISWC 2012), Boston, USA, November 12, 2012*, pages 63–77, 2012.

97. C.E.J. Kahn and D.L. Rubin. Automated semantic indexing of figure captions to improve radiology image retrieval. *Journal of the American Medical Informatics Association*, 16:280–286, 2009.

98. Giuseppe Rizzo and Raphaël Troncy. Nerd: A framework for unifying named entity recognition and disambiguation extraction tools. In *Proceedings of the Demonstrations at the 13th Conference of the European Chapter of the Association for Computational Linguistics*, EACL '12, pages 73–76, Stroudsburg, PA, USA, 2012. Association for Computational Linguistics.

99. HealthDay. Health day news. http://consumer.healthday.com/, last accessed: 14.03.2015.

100. Alan R. Aronson, Olivier Bodenreider, Dina Demner-Fushman, Kin Wah Fung, Vivian K. Lee, James G. Mork, Aurélie Névéol, Lee Peters, and Willie J. Rogers. From indexing the biomedical literature to coding clinical text: Experience with mti and machine learning approaches. In *Proceedings of the Workshop on BioNLP 2007: Biological, Translational, and Clinical Language Processing*, BioNLP '07, pages 105–112, Stroudsburg, PA, USA, 2007. Association for Computational Linguistics.

101. Oren Etzioni, Michele Banko, Stephen Soderland, and Daniel S. Weld. Open information extraction from the web. *Commun. ACM*, 51(12):68–74, December 2008.

102. Oren Etzioni, Anthony Fader, Janara Christensen, Stephen Soderland, and Mausam Mausam. Open information extraction: the second generation. In *Proceedings of the Twenty-Second international joint conference on Artificial Intelligence - Volume One*, IJCAI'11, pages 3–10. AAAI Press, 2011.

103. Fei Wu and Daniel S. Weld. Open information extraction using wikipedia. In *Proceedings of the 48th Annual Meeting of the Association for Computational Linguistics*, ACL '10, pages 118–127, Stroudsburg, PA, USA, 2010. Association for Computational Linguistics.

104. Lucia Specia and Enrico Motta. A hybrid approach for extracting semantic relations from texts. In *Proceedings of the 2nd Workshop on Ontology Learning and Population*, pages 57–64, 2006.

105. Jianhua Li Yun Niu, Xiaodan Zhu and Graeme Hirst. Analysis of polarity information in medical text. In *AMIA Annu Symp Proc. 2005*, pages 570–574, 2005.

106. Xiaodan Zhu Yun Niu and Graeme Hirst. Using outcome polarity in sentence extraction for medical question-answering. In *AMIA Annu Symp Proc. 2006*, pages 599–603, 2006.

107. Bing Liu. *Sentiment Analysis and Opinion Mining*. Synthesis Lectures on Human Language Technologies. Morgan & Claypool Publishers, 2012.
108. Minqing Hu and Bing Liu. Mining and summarizing customer reviews. In *Proceedings of the Tenth ACM SIGKDD International Conference on Knowledge Discovery and Data Mining*, KDD '04, pages 168–177, New York, NY, USA, 2004. ACM.
109. G. Mishne. Experiments with mood classification in blog posts. In *1st Workshop on Stylistic Analysis Of Text For Information Access*, 2005.
110. Matteo Baldoni, Cristina Baroglio, Viviana Patti, and Paolo Rena. From tags to emotions: Ontology-driven sentiment analysis in the social semantic web. *Intelligenza Artificiale*, 6(1):41–54, 2012.
111. Bo Pang, Lillian Lee, and Shivakumar Vaithyanathan. Thumbs up?: sentiment classification using machine learning techniques. In *Proceedings of the ACL-02 conference on Empirical methods in natural language processing - Volume 10*, EMNLP '02, pages 79–86, Stroudsburg, PA, USA, 2002. Association for Computational Linguistics.
112. Bo Pang and Lillian Lee. A sentimental education: Sentiment analysis using subjectivity summarization based on minimum cuts. In *Proceedings of the 42Nd Annual Meeting on Association for Computational Linguistics*, ACL '04, Stroudsburg, PA, USA, 2004. Association for Computational Linguistics.
113. Peter D. Turney. Thumbs up or thumbs down?: semantic orientation applied to unsupervised classification of reviews. In *Proceedings of the 40th Annual Meeting on Association for Computational Linguistics*, ACL '02, pages 417–424, Stroudsburg, PA, USA, 2002. Association for Computational Linguistics.
114. Maria Pontiki, Dimitrios Galanis, John Pavlopoulos, Haris Papageorgiou, Ion Androutsopoulos, and Suresh Manandhar. Semeval-2014 task 4: Aspect based sentiment analysis. In *Proceedings of the 8th Intern. Workshop on Semantic Evaluation (SemEval 2014)*, pages 27–35, Dublin, Ireland, August 2014.
115. K. Denecke. Are sentiwordnet scores suited for multi-domain sentiment classification? In *Digital Information Management, 2009. ICDIM 2009. Fourth International Conference on*, pages 1–6, Nov 2009.
116. A. Montejo-Ráez, E. Martínez-Cámara, M. T. Martín-Valdivia, and L. A. Ureña López. Random walk weighting over sentiwordnet for sentiment polarity detection on twitter. In *Proceedings of the 3rd Workshop in Computational Approaches to Subjectivity and Sentiment Analysis*, WASSA '12, pages 3–10, Stroudsburg, PA, USA, 2012. Association for Computational Linguistics.
117. Stefano Baccianella, Andrea Esuli, and Fabrizio Sebastiani. Sentiwordnet 3.0: An enhanced lexical resource for sentiment analysis and opinion mining. In Nicoletta Calzolari (Conference Chair), Khalid Choukri, Bente Maegaard, Joseph Mariani, Jan Odijk, Stelios Piperidis, Mike Rosner, and Daniel Tapias, editors, *Proceedings of the Seventh International Conference on Language Resources and Evaluation (LREC'10)*, Valletta, Malta, may 2010. European Language Resources Association (ELRA).
118. Alexandra Balahur, Ralf Steinberger, Mijail Alexandrov Kabadjov, Vanni Zavarella, Erik Van der Goot, Matina Halkia, Bruno Pouliquen, and Jenya Belyaeva. Sentiment analysis in the news. *CoRR*, abs/1309.6202, 2013.
119. Philip Stone. General inquirer. http://www.wjh.harvard.edu/~inquirer/, last accessed: 14.03.2015.
120. Ro Valitutti. Wordnet-affect: an affective extension of wordnet. In *In Proceedings of the 4th International Conference on Language Resources and Evaluation*, pages 1083–1086, 2004.
121. Saif M. Mohammad and Peter D. Turney. Emotions evoked by common words and phrases: Using mechanical turk to create an emotion lexicon. In *Proceedings of the NAACL HLT 2010 Workshop on Computational Approaches to Analysis and Generation of Emotion in Text*, CAAGET '10, pages 26–34, Stroudsburg, PA, USA, 2010. Association for Computational Linguistics.
122. Lingjia Deng, Yoonjung Choi, and Janyce Wiebe. Benefactive/malefactive event and writer attitude annotation. In *ACL (2)*, pages 120–125, 2013.

123. Lorraine Goeuriot, Jin-Cheon Na, Wai Yan Min Kyaing, Christopher Khoo, Yun-Ke Chang, Yin-Leng Theng, and Jung-Jae Kim. Sentiment lexicons for health-related opinion mining. In *Proceedings of the 2Nd ACM SIGHIT International Health Informatics Symposium*, IHI '12, pages 219–226, New York, NY, USA, 2012. ACM.

124. B. Ohana, B. Tierney, and S. Delany. Domain independent sentiment classification with many lexicons. In *Advanced Information Networking and Applications (WAINA), 2011 IEEE Workshops of International Conference on*, pages 632–637, March 2011.

125. Philip J. Stone and Earl B. Hunt. A computer approach to content analysis: Studies using the general inquirer system. In *Proceedings of the May 21-23, 1963, Spring Joint Computer Conference*, AFIPS '63 (Spring), pages 241–256, New York, NY, USA, 1963. ACM.

126. Grady Ward. Moby lexicon project. http://icon.shef.ac.uk/Moby, last accessed: 14.03.2015.

127. Tanveer Ali, David Schramm, Marina Sokolova, and Diana Inkpen. Can i hear you? sentiment analysis on medical forums. In *Proceedings of the Sixth International Joint Conference on Natural Language Processing*, pages 667–673, Nagoya, Japan, October 2013. Asian Federation of Natural Language Processing.

128. Lei Xia, Anna Lisa Gentile, James Munro, and José Iria. Improving patient opinion mining through multi-step classification. In Václav Matousek and Pavel Mautner, editors, *TSD*, volume 5729 of *Lecture Notes in Computer Science*, pages 70–76. Springer, 2009.

129. Jin-Cheon Na, Wai Yan Min Kyaing, Christopher S. G. Khoo, Schubert Foo, Yun-Ke Chang, and Yin Leng Theng. Sentiment classification of drug reviews using a rule-based linguistic approach. In Hsin-Hsi Chen and Gobinda Chowdhury, editors, *ICADL*, volume 7634 of *Lecture Notes in Computer Science*, pages 189–198. Springer, 2012.

130. Marina Sokolova, Stan Matwin, Yasser Jafer, and David Schramm. How joe and jane tweet about their health: Mining for personal health information on twitter. In Galia Angelova, Kalina Bontcheva, and Ruslan Mitkov, editors, *RANLP*, pages 626–632. RANLP 2011 Organising Committee / ACL, 2013.

131. P. Biyani, C. Caragea, P. Mitra, and et al. Co-training over domain-independent and domain-dependent features for sentiment analysis of an online cancer support community. In *Advances in Social Networks Analysis and Mining (ASONAM), 2013 IEEE/ACM International Conference on*, pages 413–17, 2013.

132. N. Ofek, C. Caragea, L. Rokach, P. Biyani, and et al. Improving sentiment analysis in an online cancer survivor community using dynamic sentiment lexicon. In *Social Intelligence and Technology (SOCIETY), 2013 International Conference on*, pages 109–13, 2013.

133. Phillip Smith and Mark Lee. Cross-discourse development of supervised sentiment analysis in the clinical domain. In *Proceedings of the 3rd Workshop in Computational Approaches to Subjectivity and Sentiment Analysis*, WASSA '12, pages 79–83, Stroudsburg, PA, USA, 2012. Association for Computational Linguistics.

134. H. Sharif, A. Abbasi, F. Zafar, and D. Zimbra. Detecting adverse drug reactions using a sentiment classification framework. In *Proceedings of the sixth ASE international conference on social computing (SocialCom)s*, 2014.

135. Marina Sokolova and Victoria Bobicev. What sentiments can be found in medical forums. In *Proceedings of Recent Advances in Natural Language Processing*, pages 633–639, Hissar, Bulgaria, September 2013.

136. S. Melzi, A. Abdaoui, J. Aze, S. Bringay, P. Poncelet, and F. Galtier. Patients rationale: Patient knowledge retrieval from health forums. In *Proceedings of the eTelemed 2014: Sixth Conference on eHealth, Telemedicine and Social Medicine*, pages 140–145, 2014.

137. Yun Niu, Xiaodan Zhu, Jianhua Li, and Graeme Hirst. Analysis of polarity information in medical text. In *In: Proceedings of the American Medical Informatics Association 2005 Annual Symposium*, pages 570–574, 2005.

138. Abeed Sarker, Diego Molla, and Cecile Paris. Outcome polarity identification of medical papers. In *Proceedings of the Australasian Language Technology Association Workshop 2011*, pages 105–114, Canberra, Australia, December 2011.

139. John P. Pestian, Pawel Matykiewicz, Michelle Linn-Gust, Brett South, Ozlem Uzuner, Jan Wiebe, Kevin B. Cohen, John Hurdle, and Christopher Brew. Sentiment analysis of suicide notes: A shared task. *Biomedical Informatics Insights*, 5:3–16, 01–2012.

140. Erik Cambria, Tim Benson, Chris Eckl, and Amir Hussain. Sentic proms: Application of sentic computing to the development of a novel unified framework for measuring health-care quality. *Expert Syst. Appl.*, 39(12):10533–10543, September 2012.

141. H. Liu and P. Singh. Conceptnet — a practical commonsense reasoning tool-kit. *BT Technology Journal*, 22(4):211–226, October 2004.

142. Erik Cambria, Andrew Livingstone, and Amir Hussain. The hourglass of emotions. In *Proceedings of the 2011 International Conference on Cognitive Behavioural Systems*, COST'11, pages 144–157, Berlin, Heidelberg, 2012. Springer-Verlag.

143. P. G. Mutalik, A. Deshpande, and P. M. Nadkarni. Use of general-purpose negation detection to augment concept indexing of medical documents: a quantitative study using the UMLS. *Journal of the American Medical Informatics Association : JAMIA*, 8(6):598–609, 2001.

144. Wendy Webber Chapman, Will Bridewell, Paul Hanbury, Gregory F. Cooper, and Bruce G. Buchanan. A simple algorithm for identifying negated findings and diseases in discharge summaries. *Journal of Biomedical Informatics*, 34(5):301–310, 2001.

145. Nigel Collier. Uncovering text mining: A survey of current work on web-based epidemic intelligence. *Global Public Health*, pages 731–749, 2012.

146. C. Paquet, D. Coulombier, R. Kaier, and M. Ciotti. Epidemic intelligence: a new framework for strengthening disease surveillance in europe. *Euro Surveillance*, 11(12), 2006.

147. J. P. Linge, R. Steinberger, F. Fuart, S. Bucci, J. Belyaeva, M. Gemo, D. Al-Khudhairy, R. Yangarber, and E. van der Goot. Medisys-medical information system. In *Advanced ICTs for Disaster Management and Threat Detection: Collaborative and Distributed Frameworks*. IGI Global Press, 2010.

148. P. von Etter, S. Huttunen, A. Vihavainen, M. Vuorinen, and R. Yangarber. Assessment of utility in web mining for the domain of public health. In *Proceedings of the NAACL HLT 2010 Second Louhi Workshop on Text and Data Mining of Health Documents*, pages 29–37, 2012.

149. A.F. Dugas, Y.-H. Hsieh, S.R. Levin, and et al. Google flu trends: Correlation with emergency department influenza rates and crowding metrics. *Clin Infect Dis 2012*, 54 (4):463–469.

150. S. Cook, C. Conrad, A.L. Fowlkes, and M.H. Mohebbi. Assessing google flu trends performance in the united states during the 2009 influenza virus a (h1n1) pandemic. *PLoS One 2011*, 6 (8), 2011.

151. H.A. Carneiro and E. Mylonakis. Google trends: a webbased tool for real-time surveillance of disease outbreaks. *Clin Infect Dis 2009*, 49 (10):1557–64, 2009.

152. G. Backfried, C. Schmidt, M. Pfeiffer, G. Quirchmayr, M. Glanzer, and K. Rainer. Open source intelligence for disaster management. intelligence and security informatics conference (eisic). pages 254–58, 2012.

153. Multilingual cross-domain temporal tagger heideltime, http://dbs.ifi.uni-heidelberg.de/heideltime (last access: 24.04.2013).

154. Stanford named entity recognizer, http://nlp.stanford.edu/software/crf-ner.shtml (last access: 24.04.2013).

155. Avare Stewart, Matthew Smith, and Wolfgang Nejdl. A transfer approach to detecting disease reporting events in blog social media. In *HT 2011*, pages 271–80, 2011.

156. Alessandro Moschitti, Daniele Pighin, and Roberto Basili. Semantic Role Labeling via Tree Kernel Joint Inference. In *Proceedings of the Tenth Conference on Computational Natural Language Learning (CoNLL-X)*, pages 61–68, New York City, June 2006. Association for Computational Linguistics.

157. L.C. Madoff. Promed-mail: An early warning system for emerging disease. *Clin Infect Dis 2004*, 39 (2):227–32, 2004.

158. Michael P. Coston. Avian flu diary. http://afludiary.blogspot.de/, last accessed: 14.03.2015.

159. Michael Hoehle. Surveillance: An r package for the surveillance of infectious diseases. *Computational Statistics*, 22 (4):571–82, 2007.

160. G. Rossi, L. Lampugnani, and M. Marchi. An approximate cusum procedure for surveillance of health events. *Statistics in Medicine*, 18:2111–2122, 1999.

161. P. Farrington, N. Andrews, A. Beale, and M. Catchpole. A statistical algorithm for the early detection of outbreaks of infectious disease. *J R Statist Soc A*, 159:547–563, 1996.
162. Jamila Hanan. Medworm. http://www.medworm.com/, last accessed: 14.03.2015.
163. K. Denecke. An architecture for diversity-aware search for medical web content. *Methods of Information in Medicine*, 51(6):549–56, 2012.
164. T. Vanhecke, M. Barnes, J. Zimmerman, and S. Shoichet. PubMed vs. HighWire Press: A head-to-head comparison of two medical literature search engines. *Computers in Biology and Medicine*, 37(9):1252–1258, September 2007.
165. P. Daumke, K. Marko, M. Propat, S. Schulz, and R. Klar. Biomedical information retrieval across languages. *Med Inform Internet Med*, 32(2):131–47, 2007.
166. P. Daumke, S. Schulz, M.L. Müller, W. Dzeyk, L. Prinzen, E.J. Pacheco, P.S. Cancian, P. Nohama, and K. Marko. Subword-based semantic retrieval of clinical and bibliograpic documents. *Methods Inf Med*, 49(2):141–47, 2010.
167. Martin Krallinger and Alfonso Valencia. Text-mining and information-retrieval services for molecular biology. *Genome Biology*, 6(7):224+, 2005.
168. T.G. Vit Novacek and S. Handschuh. Coraal towards deep exploitation of textual resources in life sciences. *Lecture Notes in Computer Science. Berlin/Heidelberg*, 5651/2009:206–215, 2009.
169. S. Dumais F. Radlinski. Improving personalized web search using result diversification. In *SIGIR 2006: Proceedings of the 29th annual international ACM SIGIR conference on Research and development in information retrieval. New York, USA*, pages 691–692, 2006.
170. M.A. Hearst and J.O. Pedersen. Reexamining the cluster hypothesis: scatter/gather on retrieval results. In *Proceedings of the 19th annual international ACM SIGIR conference on Research and development in information retrieval, SIGIR 1996. New York, USA*, pages 76–84, 1996.
171. D. Carmel A. Anagnostopoulos, A.Z. Broder. Sampling search-engine results. In *Proceedings of the 14th international conference on World Wide Web: New York, USA*, pages 245–256, 2005.
172. Chein-Shung Hwang and Show-Fen Lin. Hill climbing for diversity retrieval. *Computer Science and Information Engineering, World Congress on*, 5:154–158, 2009.
173. Rakesh Agrawal, Sreenivas Gollapudi, Alan Halverson, and Samuel Ieong. Diversifying search results. In *Proceedings of the Second ACM International Conference on Web Search and Data Mining*, WSDM '09, pages 5–14, New York, NY, USA, 2009. ACM.
174. Sreenivas Gollapudi and Aneesh Sharma. An axiomatic approach for result diversification. In *Proceedings of the 18th International Conference on World Wide Web*, WWW '09, pages 381–390, New York, NY, USA, 2009. ACM.
175. Enrico Minack, Gianluca Demartini, and Wolfgang Nejdl. Current approaches to search result diversification. In *Proc. of 1st Intl. Workshop on Living Web*, 2009.
176. Wisam Dakka and Panagiotis G. Ipeirotis. Automatic extraction of useful facet hierarchies from text databases. In *Proceedings of the 2008 IEEE 24th International Conference on Data Engineering*, ICDE '08, pages 466–475, Washington, DC, USA, 2008. IEEE Computer Society.
177. Marti A. Hearst. Clustering versus faceted categories for information exploration. *Commun. ACM*, 49(4):59–61, April 2006.
178. J. Diederich and W. T. Balke. Automatically created concept graphs using descriptive keywords in the medical domain. *Methods of Information in Medicine*, 47(3):241–50, 2008.
179. SJ. Darmoni, JP. Leroy, F. Baudic, M. Douyere, J. Piot, and B. Thrion. Cismef: a structured health resource guide. *Methods of Information in Medicine*, 39(1):30–35, 2000.
180. Angelos Hliaoutakis, Giannis Varelas, Euripides G. M. Petrakis, and Evangelos Milios. Medsearch: A retrieval system for medical information based on semantic similarity. In *In Proceedings of ECDL*, pages 512–515, 2006.
181. Gang Luo. Design and evaluation of the imed intelligent medical search engine. In *Proceedings of the 2009 IEEE International Conference on Data Engineering*, ICDE '09, pages 1379–1390, Washington, DC, USA, 2009. IEEE Computer Society.

182. AlchemyAPI. Alchemyapi. http://www.alchemyapi.com/, last accessed: 14.03.2015.

183. Andrea Esuli and Fabrizio Sebastiani. Sentiwordnet: A publicly available lexical resource for opinion mining. In *In Proceedings of the 5th Conference on Language Resources and Evaluation (LREC 2006)*, pages 417–422, 2006.

184. Mark Hall, Eibe Frank, Geoffrey Holmes, Bernhard Pfahringer, Peter Reutemann, and Ian H. Witten. The weka data mining software: An update. *SIGKDD Explor. Newsl.*, 11(1):10–18, November 2009.

185. Ian H. Witten and Eibe Frank. *Data Mining: Practical Machine Learning Tools and Techniques*. The Morgan Kaufmann Series in Data Management Systems. Morgan Kaufmann Publishers, San Francisco, CA, 2nd edition, 2005.

186. H. Mueller, C. Boyer, A. Gaudinat, W. Hersh, and A. Geissbuhler. Analyzing web log files of the health on the net honmedia search engine to define typical image search tasks for image retrieval evaluation. In *Stud Health Technol Inform 129 (Pt 2)*, pages 1319–1323, 2007.

187. Filip Radlinski and Nick Craswell. Comparing the sensitivity of information retrieval metrics. In *Proceedings of the 33rd International ACM SIGIR Conference on Research and Development in Information Retrieval*, SIGIR '10, pages 667–674, New York, NY, USA, 2010. ACM.

188. Kalervo Järvelin and Jaana Kekäläinen. Ir evaluation methods for retrieving highly relevant documents. In *Proceedings of the 23rd Annual International ACM SIGIR Conference on Research and Development in Information Retrieval*, SIGIR '00, pages 41–48, New York, NY, USA, 2000. ACM.

189. N.H. Shah C. Jonquet and M.A. Musen. The open biomedical annotator. In *Summit on Translat Bioinforma*, pages 56–60, 2009.

190. Tagesspiegel. Hasso-plattner-institut stoppt facebook-projekt der schufa. http://www.tagesspiegel.de/politik/datenschutz-hasso-plattner-institut-stoppt-facebook-projekt-der-schufa/6726234.html, last accessed: 14.03.2015.

191. Peter V. Conveney, Vanessa Diaz-Zuccarini, Peter Hunter, and Marco Viceconti (eds.). *Computational Biomedicine*. Oxford University Press, 2014.

192. Samuel Thompson. *The nature of Philiospophy: An Introduction*. Holt, Rinehart, and Winston, 1961.

193. I. Convery and D. Cox. A review of research ethics in internet-based research. *Practitioner Research in Higher Education*, pages 50–57, 2012.

194. IMIA. Imia social media working group. http://www.imia-medinfo.org/new2/node/289, last accessed: 14.03.2015.

195. Michal Kosinski, David Stillwell, and Thore Graepel. Private traits and attributes are predictable from digital records of human behaviour. *Proceedings of the National Academy of Sciences of the United States of America*, 2013.

196. Gunther Eysenbach and James E Till. Ethical issues in qualitative research on internet communities. *BMJ*, 323(7321):1103–1105, 2001.

197. C.S. Bond, O.H. Ahmed, M. Hind, B. Thomas, and J. Hewitt-Taylor. The conceptual and practical ethical dilemmas of using health discussion board posts as research data. *J Med Internet Res.*, 17(6), 2013.

198. Megan A. Moreno, Alison Grant, Lauren Kacvinsky, Peter Moreno, and Michael Fleming. Older adolescents' views regarding participation in facebook research. *Journal of Adolescent Health*, 51(5):439–444, 2012.

199. Michael J. Payette, Douglas Albreski, and Jane M. Grant-Kels. You'd know if you "friended" me on facebook: Legal, moral, and ethical considerations of online social media. *Journal of American Academy of Dermatology*, 69:305–7, 2013.

200. F. Gholami-Kordkheili, V. Wild, and D. Strech. The impact of social media on medical professionalism: a systematic qualitative review of challenges and opportunities. *J Med Internet Res.*, 15(8), 2013.

201. K.C. Chretien and T. Kind. Social media and clinical care: ethical, professional, and social implications. *Circulation*, pages 1413–1421, 2013.

202. J.M. Farnan, Sulmasy L. Snyder, B.K. Worster, H.K. Chaudhry, J.A. Rhyne, V.M. Arora, and et al. Online medical professionalism: Patient and public relationships: Policy statement from the american college of physicians and the federation of state medical boards. *Ann Intern Med.*, pages 620–627, 2013.

203. A. Markham and E. Buchanan. *Ethical Decision-Making and Internet Research: Recommendations from the AoIR Ethics Workin Committee.* Ethics Working Committee, 2012.

204. Medical Association. Opinion 9.124 - professionalism in the use of social media. *URL: http://www.ama-assn.org/resources/doc/code-medical-ethics/9124a.pdf (last accessed: 08.12.2013),* 2013.

205. U. Huw. Socio-economic research in the information society. *URL: http://www. respectproject.org/pubs/ethics.php (last access: 10.12.2013),* 2002.

206. H.U. Lemke and L. Berliner. Integration von informationen und cas-systemen mit einem therapy imaging and model management system (timms). In S. Eulenstein P.M. Schlag and T. Lange, editors, *Computerassistierte Chirurgie, 1. Edition,* pages 311–32. Elsevier, 2011.

207. O. Doessel. Patientenmodelle. pages 14–19, 2012.

208. L.C. van der Gaag, S. Renooij, C.L.M. Witteman, B.M.P. Aleman, and B.G. Taal. Probabilities for a probabilistic network: a case study in oesophageal cancer. *Artificial Intelligence in Medicine,* pages 123–48, 2002.

209. L. Leibovici, M. Paul, A. D. Nielsen, E. Tacconelli, and S. Andreassen. The treat project: decision support and prediction using causal probabilistic networks. *International Journal of Antimicrobial Agents,* 30 (Supplement 1):93–102, 2007.

210. K. Denecke. Model-based decision support: Requirements and future for its application in surgery. *Biomedical Engineering/Biomedizinische Technik, Biomed Tech,* 56 (Suppl 1), 2013.

211. Agnieszka Oniko and Marek J. Druzdzel. Impact of precision of bayesian network parameters on accuracy of medical diagnostic systems. *Artif. Intell. Med.,* 57(3):197–206, March 2013.

212. M. Cypko, M. Stoehr, K. Denecke, A. Dietz, and H.U. Lemke. User interaction with mebns for large patient-specific treatment decision models with an example for laryngeal cancer. *Int J CARS, Volume 9 (Suppl 1),* 2014.

213. Gregory F. Cooper and Edward Herskovits. A bayesian method for the induction of probabilistic networks from data. In *MACHINE LEARNING,* pages 309–347, 1992.

214. Peter Antal, Geert Fannes, Dirk Timmerman, Yves Moreau, and Bart De Moor. Using literature and data to learn bayesian networks as clinical models of ovarian tumors. *Artificial Intelligence in Medicine,* 30(3):257–281, 2004.

215. O.W. Tchami, M-C. L'Homme, and N. Grabar. Discovering semantic frames for a contrastive study of verbs in medical corpora. *Terminologie Intelligence Artificielle (TIA),* 2013.

216. Y. Wang, S. Pakhomov, N.E. Burkart, J.O. Ryan, and G.B. Melton. A study of actions in operative notes. In *AMIA Annu Symp Proc.,* pages 1431–40, 2012.

217. O. Patterson and J.F. Hurdle. Document clustering of clinical narratives: a systematic study of clinical sublanguages. *AMIA Annu Symp Proc.,* pages 1099–1107, 2011.

218. E. Miscin. Use of corpus analysis tools in medical corpus processing. *INFuture2013: "Information Governance",* pages 187–196, 2013.

219. Andreas M. Kaplan and Michael Haenlein. Users of the world, unite! the challenges and opportunities of social media. *Business Horizons,* 53(1):59–68, 2010.

Index

Printed in the United States
By Bookmasters